If a doctor said to you, "I'm sorry, it's canc reading this very well researched book, m I'd take it from there and start to ask the ri people and make sure to make "my own" r̶i̶g̶h̶t̶ ̶d̶e̶c̶i̶s̶i̶o̶n̶s̶ ̶r̶e̶g̶a̶r̶d̶i̶n̶g̶ ̶h̶o̶w̶ ̶t̶o̶ proceed.

This is exactly what this book is all about. Please make sure you do not miss a single word as you go through it.

It is very evident that Wanda St. Hilaire is a wise and loving person and she has made a huge effort to bring to everyone a "very" holistic approach to help us travel down the highway of cancer whether we are patients or friends.

Wanda's generosity becomes evident in this encyclopedic dictionary that contains, not only personal experiences and a guideline to therapies, but also a listing of outstanding clinics that have achieved very good results.

Congratulations Wanda for this masterpiece and I hope that millions of readers make the most out of it.

Good health to all of you.

—Dr. Raymond Hilu
Clinica Hilu, Spain

"I'M SORRY, IT'S CANCER", by Wanda St. Hilaire is a brilliantly written road map to navigating the realm of oncology. Ms. St. Hilaire addresses fundamental issues challenging everyone during their oncologic journey. These issues should be, but are not, addressed by oncologists. In fact, oncology refuses to recognize these issues as variables, which alter your outcome. The outline contained within this work is essential for anyone desiring to regain a cancer free status. If your goal is to achieve optimal health, free from cancer, then this book is an excellent resource.

—Carlos M. Garcia, M.D.
Medical Director at Utopia Wellness
Florida, USA

Wanda's book, *What To Do After "I'm sorry, it's cancer."* is one of the best books I have come across during my 37 years of being a physician dealing with natural methods to try to help patients with cancer.

The research she did for this book is "amazing" … I will recommend it to all my patients who suffer from this terrible disease.

—Dr. Jose Luis Romo Razo M.D.
Puerto Vallarta, Mexico

I have read *What To Do After "I'm sorry, it's cancer."* and love it. It is very warm and right from your heart. I really think this will be a great benefit for folks going through the cancer experience. So many emotions course through our minds at the speed of light when we hear that we have cancer. It can be too much to process let alone to know the right questions to ask. There is so much fear attached to those words and the treatment, ugh … that's another overwhelming process. Without experience I honestly don't know how people do it. This is why your experience will be so helpful in guiding them. I highly recommend your book for those who are facing the cancer experience!

—Valerie Warwick, RN, OCN, CMS, CLT
(Oncology/Chemotherapy Nurse)
Cancer Coach, Founder of My Wellness Tutor
Hawaii, USA

Wanda's heartfelt book is like a conversation with a trusted friend who's been there, done that. She guides the reader gently through the initial shock of a cancer diagnosis, and then offers a range of suggestions for working through options, in both traditional and complementary medicine and self-care. This is one woman's journey through breast cancer, made extraordinary by her willingness to share it with others who may be navigating a similar path.

—Wings of Hope Foundation
Calgary, Canada

This is a profound book written with passion and love. St. Hilaire finds a way to develop intimacy and frankness with the reader through this journey. This book opens the doors to many new possibilities for those willing to learn and delivers well-researched and practical advice.

The reader is left feeling the warmth of having sunk into a couch with a trusted friend to have a serious conversation about life. Congratulations to Wanda for delivering her wealth of knowledge and experience in a very accessible and thorough manner. This book succeeds in removing fear from cancer and leading the reader towards high ground.

I wish all those who read this book the very best in their journey towards health and happiness.

–Dr. Dustin Whitney, DC.
Calgary, Alberta, Canada

Wanda St. Hilaire's book is a fabulous tool for those affected by cancer. The initial shock of the big "C" washes over every patient, leaving them overwhelmed and terrified. They forget what questions to ask and their thoughts become muddled when they sit in front of the doctor. This book navigates the reader through a lot of cancer research, allowing the diagnosed to have greater understanding and insight during their own journey.

What To Do After "I'm sorry, it's cancer." also answers many questions that race through each and every patient and caregiver's mind. It gives hope for a light at the end of the tunnel, and provides options for those affected by this terrible disease. It is a "must read" for everyone. Thank you Wanda for sharing your research and wisdom!

—Dr. Janelle Murphy, ND
Calgary, Alberta, Canada

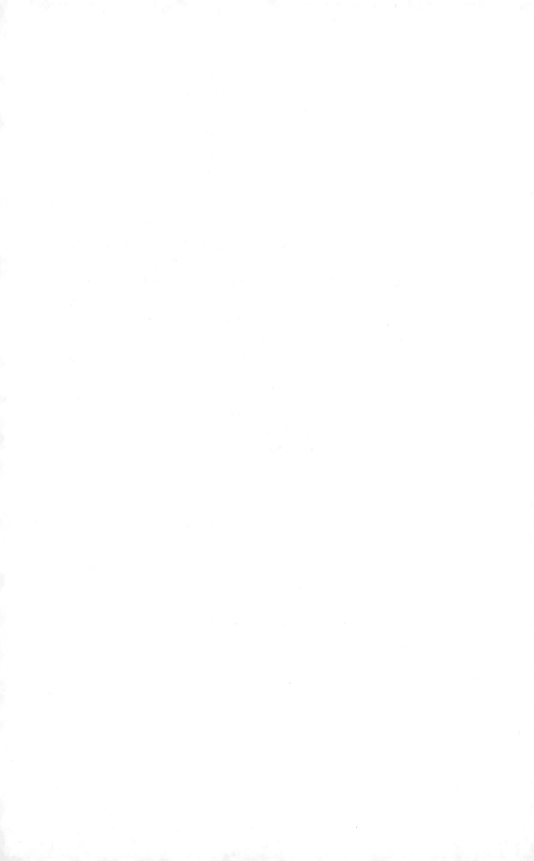

WHAT TO DO AFTER

"I'M SORRY, IT'S CANCER."

AN EXCEPTIONAL GUIDEBOOK FOR NAVIGATING YOUR WAY TO HEALTH AND HAPPINESS

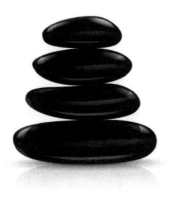

WANDA ST. HILAIRE

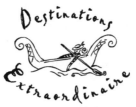

CALGARY, ALBERTA

What To Do After "I'm sorry, it's cancer."
An Exceptional Guidebook for Navigating Your Way to Health and Happiness
Copyright © 2017 Wanda St. Hilaire. All Rights Reserved.

Published by
Destinations Extraordinaire
1103-339 10 Ave SE
Calgary, AB, T2G 0W2
Canada

ISBN: 978-1-894331-14-2

Cover art by Ding Sidek
Cover Design and Book Layout by Ryan Fitzgerald
Pheasant Illustration © www.gograph.com / basel101658
(http://www.gograph.com/search/artist/basel101658)
Spa stones image is licensed by www.rfclipart.com / Vasyl Duda
(https://rfclipart.com/user/dvarg)

www.imsorryitscancer.com
www.writewaycafe.com
www.wandasthilaire.com

Edition: June 2017

This book is dedicated with love to my soul sister, Lynnette, and tied to a prayer that something in these pages will lead her to a spontaneous remission.

♥

It was the best of times, it was the worst of times, it was the age of wisdom, it was the age of foolishness, it was the epoch of belief, it was the epoch of incredulity, it was the season of Light, it was the season of Darkness, it was the spring of hope, it was the winter of despair, we had everything before us, we had nothing before us, we were all going direct to heaven, we were all going direct the other way...
—Charles Dickens
A Tale of Two Cities

TABLE OF CONTENTS

INTRODUCTION – WHY ANOTHER CANCER BOOK? .xv

THE C WORD: DECISIONS   1
1. STOP. BREATHE. 3
2. SHARING 7
3. RESEARCH 9
4. THE DOCTORS 13
5. CONVENTIONAL MEDICINE 19
6. INTEGRATIVE AND COMPLEMENTARY MEDICINE. 29
7. IT *IS* ALL ABOUT YOU RIGHT NOW 49
8. MAKE AN INTEGRATIVE WELLNESS AND SELF-CARE PLAN 53
9. WORK. 57
10. FINANCES 59
11. TEAM HEAL 61
12. CONNECTION. GROUPS. THERAPY. 65
    BLOG: NO MAN'S AN ISLAND 68
13. NUTRITION MATTERS. PERIOD. 73
14. THE ANTIDOTE TO FEAR IS TRUST 83
    BLOG: THE EENSY WEENSY SPIDER 84
15. STRESS. 89
    BLOG: LIGHTEN UP, FRANCIS!. 94
16. NATURE. 97
    BLOG: THE LOST ART 100
17. MORALE BOOSTING: THINK OUTSIDE THE BUN 105
18. FILL YOUR MIND WITH POSSIBILITY 109
    BLOG: THE ART OF IMPOSSIBILITY. 112
19. NEGATIVITY FASTING. 117
20. WHY ME?. 121
    BLOG: THE WORST BEST THINGS IN LIFE 123
21. DO WHAT YOU LOVE. 127
    BLOG: THE FEEDING AND WATERING OF A SOUL 130
22. SELF-TALK 135
    BLOG: THE TAMING OF THE TWERP. 139
23. ATTITUDE 145
24. GRATITUDE. 149
    BLOG: GRATITUDE AND TASTY TURKEYS 151

DOWN THE RABBIT HOLE   155
25. A PIVOTAL MOMENT. 157
    BLOG: THE TIME OF YOUR LIFE. 159
26. SPIRITUALITY 163
27. MEDITATION AND MINDFULNESS. 165
    BLOG: TO BE OR NOT TO BE. 167

28. EFT TAPPING 171
29. VISUALIZATION 173
30. CANCER AS A LIFESTYLE—NOT 177
31. RANDOM ACTS OF KINDNESS 181
    BLOG: PREMEDITATED ACTS OF KINDNESS AND PURPOSE DRIVEN BEAUTY . . 182
32. LIVING LIFE BY HEART 189
33. WHAT'S EATING YOU? 193
    BLOG: WHAT IF? 201
34. FORGIVE 205
35. SELF-WORTH 209
    BLOG: LET IT GO 212
36. TO THINE OWN SELF BE TRUE 217
    BLOG: A DOLPHIN IN THE SNOW 220
37. DEPRESSION 225
38. PURPOSE 229
    BLOG: THE YELLOW BRICK PATH TO YOUR PURPOSE 231
39. MOVEMENT, MUSIC, AND THE BREATH 235
    BLOG: THE SWEET, SWEET SOUND OF MUSIC 238
40. LOVE YOURSELF 243
    BLOG: HOW DO I LOVE THEE? 246
41. VULNERABILITY 251
    BLOG: THE UPSIDE OF VULNERABILITY 254

ALL THE WAY DOWN THE RABBIT HOLE   259
42. EPIGENETICS 261
43. QUANTUM HEALING 265
    BLOG: THE RABBIT HOLE OF REINVENTING YOURSELF 269
44. THE MAGICAL 273
    BLOG: PRACTICAL EVERYDAY MAGIC 275
45. THE MYSTICAL 279
    BLOG: SUBTLE SIGNS AND SWEET SERENDIPITY 281
46. THE MIRACULOUS 287
47. I HOPE YOU DANCE 291

MY GRATITUDE 295
THE REINVENT CANCER PROJECT 297
RESOURCES 299
ABOUT THE AUTHOR 303

DISCLOSURE

The opinions expressed in this book are ones that have been formed from two firsthand experiences of breast cancer and years of research. I do not profess to be an expert on cancer and the material in this book is to be taken solely as advisory. By sharing information that people diagnosed with cancer may not have access to, I offer to serve.

This book is not intended for the treatment or prevention of any disease, nor as a substitute for medical treatment, nor as an alternative to medical advice. Use of any recommendations included in this book is the choice of the individual and all readers assume full responsibility for the options they make on their cancer journey. If medical advice is required, readers should seek it from the appropriate medical professional.

I have no affiliation to any person, place, or thing I have covered in this book.

Wanda St. Hilaire

Why Another Cancer Book?
(Pertinent "Read-Me" Intro)

"No one is immune—life happens."
—Les Brown
World-class motivational speaker and cancer survivor

In early 2010 I made plans to celebrate—in a big way. It was to be my 20th anniversary of living cancer-free. My best friend had also gone through breast cancer and was at the five-year mark. We had talked about Italy for a decade, so we finally booked a flight to Rome for a 'celebration of life' trip in autumn. I was ecstatic.

Two weeks later, I went out on a dinner date with a new suitor, after which he kissed me goodnight at the door. Later, as I tucked myself into bed, it struck me that I hadn't done a breast exam in a while. To my utter horror, I found a large lump in my left breast.

It was cancer.

There are few words in the Western world that evoke more terror than, *"I'm sorry, it's cancer."* Until you have heard that brief, heartbreaking sentence, you cannot know the tsunami-like impact on your psyche—and on your entire existence.

To say I was shocked the second time around, after twenty years of good health under my belt, is an understatement. I knew I was not emotionally or physically prepared for what lay ahead of me, so I opted to go to Mexico to boost my immunity with chelation and complementary therapies. I walked the shoreline and sat by the ocean to quell my spirit. I returned home and had a lumpectomy and radiation, completing treatments September 2010.

We are bombarded by the efforts of the war on cancer: the race for a cure, cancer awareness, cancer fundraisers, and pink ribbon campaigns on every product imaginable. We have seen people around us suffer deeply. We are advised, informed, and have outright seen that cancer kills.

Living under this black cloud, we are unaware that many cultures view cancer quite differently than we do in North America. Others find it is much less menacing, far more natural, and it is therefore handled in a calm manner with spiritual undertones. In some places, cancer is considered an imbalance to be balanced and the focus is on becoming stronger and better than before.

I know all too well the abject fear and acute sense of overwhelm that follows a diagnosis of cancer and, with that in mind, I have distilled a mountain of information into bite-sized, easy to digest chapters. However, I realize the first segment of this book is heavy. But please stick with me; I have purposefully arranged it this way to give you the hard information first so that you can make educated decisions. After the dry, harsh part comes the softer soul food—the essential piece that is so often missed in a cancer healing quest.

I am not a health professional. I am a writer and a two-time cancer survivor with a penchant for learning. My motive for the extensive research I have done over the past twenty-five years regarding the body, the mind, and spirituality is to understand why we get the results we get in our lives with our health and our overall success and happiness levels. I value truth and fairness and endeavor to be a catalyst for change.

I had been terribly blocked on a travel memoir I was writing when early one winter morning I was awakened from my sleep by a loud pronouncement in in my mind:

You are writing a book about cancer.

It was as though I had been abruptly handed an "assignment." I argued. I'd had no previous notions to write about cancer and did not want to tackle it. I refused. It would be neither fun nor sexy—I write travel memoir and inspirational pieces.

But the subsequent message bleated resolutely:

You *will* write it.

I reluctantly began an outline; surprisingly the content flowed. This project pulled me from what I would classify as a five-year post cancer funk that was exacerbated by an epic flood (a natural disaster), one that ripped its way through my life just as I was rebounding.

The process of writing this book became enjoyable because I recognized that what I have learned is a pocket of much-needed information for those diagnosed. This book holds wisdom that grew through many kick-ass challenges, and material from many years of study and research. Developing and composing the book has given my life purpose in a way I had not previously considered, and this undertaking gives meaning and light to times of despair and darkness.

Where the book lands is not my business. I only knew that I had to write it. As I wrote, my main mission became clear: to help you, the diagnosed, make fully informed decisions that will best support you to renewed health and assist you in discovering a quality of life that is better than before. My deepest wish is that your suffering is minimized. In addition, I want to remind you that impossible things happen every day.

I always savor the allegorical stories in a non-fiction book because they help me assimilate information. There is a North American Native quote that sums up the style of this book: *"Tell me a fact and I'll listen, tell me a truth and I'll hear, but tell me a story and it will live in my heart forever."*

At the end of various chapters you will find a story from my blog, Life by Heart. I was inspired to create this blog after my second diagnosis. Selected posts illustrate the preceding chapter and are intended to lighten your burden and soothe your heart. If you are not a story-loving type of person, just skip past them.

It is highly improbable that all of what is contained in this book will resonate with you. Our beliefs and indoctrination determine our neutrality or openness to new concepts, so there may be ideas you are not ready to hear. I can attest to the fact that humans are resistant to change, but I am certain that there will be at least one thing in this book that will make your journey easier. With that in mind, I will have accomplished the task I was "assigned."

Above all, be ever so gentle with yourself. Do not do anything that I, or that anyone suggests—doctors included—if it does not feel good or right to you at a deep gut level. Go to your internal guidance system first, your all-knowing heart and intuition, to make the important decisions. There are a thousand things you can do to help heal cancer. Do what is right for you.

One thing that I believe is a non-optional part of a cancer journey is the absolute necessity to love yourself through the process. Say it out loud. I love you [your name]. Repeat it many times daily. Self-love is the best medicine in the world.

I send *my* love and 100,000 angels to each of you. I wish for you the very best on your path to wellness.

May the Force be with you.

P.S. I invite you to visit the links listed in this book. I have spent innumerable hours sourcing interesting stories, music, and valuable information that will move you, astound you, and assist you.

The C Word: Decisions

1

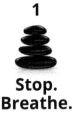

Stop.
Breathe.

"Fear of a name increases fear of the thing itself."
—J.K. Rowling
Harry Potter and the Philosopher's Stone

I know. It hit you physically, like a blow. Someplace in your body, everything froze or turned upside down. One day you were a healthy human being nonchalantly going through the motions of your life, and the next day, you were broadsided. Life looks normal on the outside, but it is not on the inside.

The most common reaction to a cancer diagnosis is to panic first, breathe later. Much later. Next, there is the "get-it-out-*now*!" response and you are tossed into the maelstrom of the cancer cog.

When I say breathe, I literally mean, *breathe*. Sit down someplace quiet and take deep, slow breaths, breathing through your nose and blowing out of your mouth. Fill your diaphragm and belly. Whenever you feel like your head is going to explode, sit down and take ten deep breaths.

Right now you are overwhelmed and most likely confused. It is hard to make good decisions when you are panicked. And it is difficult to listen. As challenging as it is to do, it will serve you both in the short and long term to be still and go within. Listen to what your gut instincts are telling you.

Right after I found a lump in my breast for the second time, I was away working in the city where my first cancer had occurred. I booked an emergency mammogram and after the technician was done, she asked me to stay. A doctor, with little to no bedside manner, came in to speak with me. She reiterated, *"This is serious,"* numerous times as she berated me for not agreeing to an immediate ultrasound.

But my hearing became impaired; it was as though I was listening to her speak in slow motion from the bottom of a barrel. I was in a state of shock and I had clients to see in a small town on my way home. My mind and body were reeling and all I wanted to do was get out of that cancer institution, fast.

I don't remember the drive down the highway. My head was turbulent and my thoughts darted from one to another, but I do recall as I turned the corner onto a rural artery, that I looked out into a vast snow-covered field and saw a coyote skulking across the stark plain. As I drove into the frozen landscape, my breathing shifted and my focus moved from my whirling thoughts down to my heart. I became calm. Then I asked myself the hard question:

If this is cancer again, what are you going to do?

Answers flashed into my mind immediately, with crisp clarity.

Firstly, I will go to Mexico for natural treatments to strengthen my body. I will walk in nature and sit ocean-side to calm my spirit and prepare for what lies ahead.

Secondly, I will spend time healing in the beauty of the Okanagan Valley with my sister. She is my source of unconditional love and will hold no opinions or judgments about what I need or what I do.

Thirdly, I will go to Italy with my best friend, come hell or high water.

In that moment, I decided that I would keenly listen to my heart and my intuition on this journey. I would do cancer my way and, older and wiser, I would be firm in making decisions with my body.

When I met with the surgeon, I told him my plan to spend a month pre-surgery in Mexico to prepare emotionally and to get immune-boosting complementary treatments. I asked if he saw a problem with the time lag. Even though he did not have any knowledge of the protocols I would be using, and could not endorse them, based on my type of cancer, he foresaw no issues and we scheduled the surgery for six weeks later.

The medical system creates a sense of urgency, however, we do not need to fly into panic mode and a "get it out now!" mentality. Being whisked into the cancer process and thrown into surgery instantaneously leaves you no time to compose and prepare. Of course, if it is extremely aggressive, that needs to be factored in; however, cancer can take years to develop into a tumor. No matter the situation, you have *some* time to stop, regroup, and research. You will need a lot of energy to heal; hurling yourself into a medical labyrinth is draining and confusing, to say the least.

You have answers within. Stop to listen to the responses your intuition will give you about what is best for your body in regard to recommendations for surgery, treatments, and whatever is paramount for your ultimate recovery. Note the difference between response and reaction. Before you charge off in a frenzy to kill cancer, spend time alone in reflection so that you can hear yourself away from the noise of everyone else's opinions and advice.

I am going to be raw and candid. The source of your fear is the elephant in the room. Nobody wants to say it. You may feel like running away in terror or curling up and hiding when you think about it. We have been pummeled with images of people looking like Holocaust victims lumbering to a slow and painful demise. We have had firsthand experience of friends or family who have deteriorated or passed. *We don't want to suffer.*

In my own experience of cancer, and in further research for this book, I have learned about the multitude of alternatives to that bleak and painful picture. In the writing of this book, the heavy cloud of fear in my own mind has lifted.

I recommend this simple breathing exercise, three times per day, to help clear anxiety and oxygenate your body: Breathe deeply through your nose. Hold for a count to ten. Exhale intensely through your mouth. Repeat ten times.

Take a time out. Assess where you are right now physically, emotionally, spiritually, and financially. Do your research. After you are informed, in the quietest moment, ask your higher self:

> *Why am I sick?*
> *What will heal me?*

Do not ignore your instinct. Seek what is best for you. No two humans are alike and you are the expert of your body. Proceed accordingly.

2

Sharing

"If you reveal your secrets to the wind, you should not blame the wind for revealing them to the trees."
—Khalil Gibran

Ensure people know where you stand in regard to your preference for privacy. Personally, I like and want support. The more well-wishers and prayers the better. But you may not want friends and family plastering your news all over Facebook, or someone in management spreading the information throughout the company. It's vital to be clear about your wishes before a well-meaning someone sends out a missive.

As you go through this passage, you may choose to send group emails to friends and family with updates to keep things simple instead of constantly repeating yourself to the point of exhaustion. You can also ask a friend or family member to do so for you.

I highly recommend discretion when sharing your decisions in regards to your treatments and wellness plan. It is startling how even complete strangers will tell you what to do without consideration for your freedom to choose—even if they have never been through cancer themselves. A simple, 'I prefer not to discuss my regimen' works well. My experience is that harsh opinions can knock you out of equilibrium and will seed more doubt and fear. Manage your thoughts and delete the rigid viewpoints of others if they make you feel disempowered or wrong for your decisions.

It is wonderful that people may want to help by sending you articles they have read and information on treatments they have discovered. Be open. There are cutting-edge approaches frequently emerging from different corners of the globe. Accept the information; you never know what it may offer. If you are too distracted to process or research what you have been given, assign the task to a friend or family member and ask for a condensed version. If you find a suitable volunteer, provide their email address instead of yours for the sole purpose of incoming information friends want to share.

Be careful not to isolate out of a sense of stoicism or of hyper-privacy. People need people, especially at times of crisis and it is people who will carry you through with their kindness, care, love, and prayers.

3

Research

"Cancer is a symptom of an imbalance in our bodies where the immune system has been overwhelmed temporarily. We can restore that almost entirely with almost any kind of cancer. But, we have to be aware of what this is in order to deal with it."
—Bill Henderson
Cure Your Cancer

Knowledge is empowerment. If you have not already done so, research your diagnosis. If it is too overwhelming for you, have someone who is skilled at fact-finding do it for you. It is important that you have a clear understanding of your options. Some hospitals use treatments and protocols that are decades old—some sixty years. Other regions may offer more progressive alternatives.

Recognize that medicine does not have all of the answers. The first time I was diagnosed with breast cancer, a lumpectomy, lymph node resection, and radiation was recommended. The radiation was full breast and armpit, five days a week, for five weeks. The lymph nodes were clean and clear of cancer, so chemotherapy was not mentioned.

With the second diagnosis, the same protocol was initially recommended. Twenty years later and *billions* of dollars in research money poured into breast cancer and the same treatment was being offered? I questioned this and was shocked that procedures for breast cancer were no further ahead (detection remains the same breast crushing mammogramic technology as well). I decided that unless there was something leading edge available in radiation treatments, I would decline.

My oncologist revealed that a clinical test study of 3000+ women had just been completed and I was allowed to opt for the new therapy. I could have localized (focused around the tumor site) radiation instead of full breast. It would be only five days, but twice a day with an intensified dosage.

Because of my radiation experience, I still thought long and hard about whether or not to do it. My gut said that twice a day would be too intense. I asked about the possibility of one dose per day. That option was not available. Based on my type and stage of cancer, my oncologist said that there was a 30% chance I needed the radiation, but they had no way to know if I was in the 30% group who would fare better with treatment or the 70% group who would not benefit from radiation due to various factors that are difficult to accurately determine.

Six years later, I learned that the standard radiation protocol for breast cancer is no longer 5 weeks, but 3 ½ weeks. I have also discovered that the localized 5-day protocol I did choose has been halted. It is under review and, if offered again, it will be only once a day at a less intense dosage. This is due to the cosmetic damage it causes to the breast. Of note, the radiation I had in 2010 caused ridges of hardened scar tissue in my left breast and chest muscle. I had painful physiotherapy sessions to break down the scar, but it didn't remedy the situation. I had intuited the dosage would be too strong, but in the end, I made a fear-based decision.

I am currently working with a biodynamic craniosacral practitioner to repair the tissue damage. After six sessions, the scarring in the breast tissue is essentially gone and the breast is soft. So far, the chest muscle is still hardened. My craniosacral practitioner is a seasoned ultrasound technician and we discussed the reason it took a couple of years for both breasts to "settle" and reveal noticeable dips in the fullness. She divulged that it is because gradually the healthy fat tissue that has been damaged by radiation shrivels and dies.

The best type of research is speaking with survivors who have been though the exact type of cancer you have been diagnosed with. Ask a cancer support group to connect you with someone. Most survivors are happy to help. You will be able to learn firsthand what the surgery and treatments were like, the impact and ramifications, tips for coping, and if that person would do things any differently in hindsight. Do take into consideration that everyone has a unique perspective on the process.

You have likely seen those frightening ads on TV with the subsequent catalog of contraindications. Do not blindly take prescriptions without researching potential side effects and irreversible damage to your body or mental faculties.

Scientific medicine is designed to be updated as new information is available. Unfortunately, Big Pharma, politics, and profit have appropriated that model. That is why you may find information on new, alternative, and advanced cures in your research that are not available at your oncology center.

In Canada, cost effectiveness for cancer health care is a significant factor as well. If you wish to try new therapies, you may need to travel, and you will usually be required to pay out of pocket. I implore you to see the value of investing in your health and ultimately, your life.

Beware that some medical sites and Wikipedia data are seeded by the pharmaceutical industry with misinformation about natural supplementation; so dig deep for reputable data. After you have done some research, write a list and take it with you to your appointments. Studies show that people who take charge of their own health have better results than those who take a passive approach and allow doctors to make all of their decisions.

4

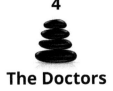

The Doctors

"The greatest mistake in the treatment of diseases is that there are physicians for the body and physicians for the soul, although the two cannot be separated."
—Plato

Life changes at warp speed upon a cancer diagnosis. You will be thrown into a maze of medical jargon, doctors, specialists, and tests. You may be assigned a surgeon and an oncologist. Remember that you have a right to choose the doctors best suited to your needs and temperament.

Before you see the doctors, sit in quietude or meditation to calm yourself. This will help you from becoming overly emotional during appointments. I cannot emphasize strongly enough the importance of getting still and centered before making life-altering decisions.

If you have done research ahead of your appointment, print off any information that you wish to discuss. Be sure to write down everything or you will never remember what you've been told. Jot notes about what the doctors say or, better still, have someone else do so for you. The latter is highly recommended. If you have an open-minded loved one who will scribe and help you project manage your diagnosis and care, you will find the journey much lighter. You can also make a request to record the appointment on your phone so that you can go over the information later (some doctors may not agree to this for legal reasons).

Be completely honest with your doctors. Do not withhold important details about your habits and lifestyle. If you drink three glasses of wine a day, say so. Offer as much pertinent information and minute specifics about any pain or progression of the condition. Yes or no answers are not enough. Let go of embarrassment; you need to reveal the whole truth to get the best possible care.

During my first go 'round with breast cancer, I made sure my surgeon understood that I was still very young and that my breasts were important to me. I did not want unnecessary nerve damage and I wanted him to take good care with the aesthetics. If such things are important to you, you need to express them. Some surgeons are only concerned with getting the tumor out and have little interest in how you will look or feel afterward. I have seen massive and deep scars on women with pea-sized tumors because they did not think they needed, or had the right, to express their requirements. If your surgeon feels you are being ridiculous, request another.

If surgery is recommended, ask *exactly* what the effects will be after the procedure. A friend had radical cancer surgery and one of the grossly unpleasant side effects was never mentioned. Had she known, she may not have had the surgery. Will there be infertility or impotence? Will you be thrown into a premature menopause? Will you have a loss of taste or smell? Will there be permanent nerve damage and a loss of sensation? Ask how your quality of life will be affected.

A surgeon's number one goal is to remove all of the cancer and its margins—which is vital—but it is you who will live with the effects, sometimes permanently. Do not let confusion or fear numb you from asking questions.

In Canada, a triage nurse at the local cancer center will assign you an oncologist. Both times I spoke to the triage nurse *before* I was assigned. I wanted a progressive oncologist who was comfortable with a patient who'd have a slew of ongoing questions; I needed someone who respected that I was in control of my own integrative wellness plan.

The first time, the nurse completely understood and assigned the perfect doctor for me. My oncologist was a brilliant woman who openly welcomed my questions. She was a cheerleader for my healing, and completely open to the complementary medicine that I was prescribed by a reputable naturopathic clinic.

The second time, the triage nurse told me that all of the doctors were equally qualified. I pressed further and reiterated my needs. She conceded that there were two or three oncologists who fit my requirements, and she placed me with an intuitive doctor who was extremely patient with my barrage of questions and concerns based on my previous experience of cancer. My oncologist that second time around truly listened and heard me. She valued my individuality and was genuinely interested in my personal life; we discussed both my challenges and my triumphs. She was fully supportive of my decision about radiation either way, did not use scare tactics, and understood my fears.

This is an emotionally charged and stressful process and you can hand-pick the right oncologist for you.

You may encounter doctors with students tailing them into your appointments for training purposes. Students do need to learn, but if you are uncomfortable with them participating in your examinations, say so. You are not required to have them present.

During my first radiation experience, I made a request for all-female technician teams to handle the procedure. At that point in time, a breast cancer patient was literally screwed to a table in a clear plastic mold with one arm around her ear. I was not comfortable being topless while affixed to a table with men in the room. The first day a male technician walked in and I explained the instructions I'd given to the oncologist. He became rude and insolent with a lot of push back, but I did not relent. I was going to be in that position many times over a five-week period and I deserved to have my wishes respected. (For the record, the three female techs in the room loudly applauded my rebuttal and high-fived me after he left.)

I recall the huge *Star Wars*-like room that I was placed in for the configuration of the radiation treatments (it has changed somewhat since then). There were two technicians and my oncologist working on the simulation, but as I lay there (again topless), an assorted group of techs and nurses were passing in and out of the room. I became increasingly uncomfortable and finally asked a random visitor why he was there. He said he had to ask my oncologist a question. I asked anyone who wasn't involved with the procedure to leave immediately.

All those present appeared shocked, but I was unyielding. They may see 200 breasts a day, but I do not expose mine 200 times a day. Privacy is a right. It was mine, and it is yours. A cancer diagnosis does not require any one to give up their rights to an opinion, a request, or privacy.

In the world of cancer, doctors are prone to quoting statistical odds for your survival. Please remember, these are statistics. The variables are astronomical. Who really knows what a patient does when they finish treatments? Are they smoking? Doing recreational drugs or over-medicating? Are they in a toxic marriage? Do they exercise? Do they eat excessive amounts of processed food or energy drinks? Are they constantly in stress mode or in a state of anger? Do they hate their jobs or even their lives?

It is important to understand that the rate of survival you will be given is based *only* on conventional treatments, not the myriad complementary options you can engage in your healing journey. We each have unique chemistry. No one can accurately determine your survival rate if you use a holistic approach and no one can precisely predict time related to conventional treatment either. Do not get lost in the diagnosis, the medicine, or in the data about what happened to somebody else.

Please understand that an oncologist will give people with certain types and stages of cancer a low chance of survival based on conventional medicine. In some alternative/complementary clinics, the success rates observed are much higher and there are cases of remissions and cures that are unheard of in traditional medicine.

The most proactive way to proceed is to understand the conventional treatments available and address the whole system: spiritual, emotional, psychological, nutritional, detoxification, energy balancing, and immune boosting. Exercise your right to consider and investigate options.

This moment is of critical importance. Can you decide, with conviction, not to allow anyone to predict your future? Can you suspend disbelief and focus on possibility? Do not let anyone brand you with fear. Mind/body medicine is growing in exponential leaps. Without explanation or statistical proof, cancer can go into remission, idleness, or vanish. Traditional medicine is resistant, because of rigid indoctrination, but it is shifting. Realize that the time lag for innovation in research and implementation can take more than fifteen years to hit mainstream medicine.

A perfect example of medical postponement, perhaps even obstinacy, is in the treatment of ulcers. For decades ulcers were treated with antacid-type remedies and prolonged, stringent, and bland diets and, as the condition painfully progressed, radical surgery that left people permanently scarred and in pain.

An internist, Barry Marshall, began working with Robin Warren on the theory that bacteria caused ulcers. Marshall and Warren traced ulcers, and stomach cancer, to gut infection. The proposed cure: antibiotics. But, as is all too often the case in medicine, Marshall was ridiculed by his peers for his discovery and conclusions.

Unable to experiment on humans, Marshall took drastic measures to prove his point; he drank a broth with H. pylori from an infected patient. Then, as predicted, he developed gastritis, the precursor to ulcers. He proved unequivocally that the H. pylori bacterium was the cause of ulcers. His recommendation for a 'cure' was spot-on: antibiotics.

Yet it took most endocrinologists 10 to 15 years to accept the information and adopt antibiotics as the prescribed cure. It was a case of sheer stubbornness, adherence to paradigms, and closed minds. The protocol to treat ulcers has only become mainstream since 2012.

In 2005, Marshall and Warren won the 2005 Nobel Peace Prize for their findings. People suffer and people die unnecessarily because of ego and tunnel vision.

Many doctors are in the biz because they are compassionate and want to help people heal. But, if for any reason you do not feel respected or heard, move on. If you want a second opinion, get one. If anyone bullies you because you feel another opinion is required, don't succumb to pressure. A doctor who forces his or her recommendations on you and does not consider your concerns or questions is not a sign of a future collaborative partnership in your health. A good relationship with an empathetic doctor who believes in you is important for your recovery and healing.

An acquaintance recently disclosed a notification he had received from his physician. He had been sent a registered letter of dismissal because he had questioned his doctor about the prescriptions he'd been given that had caused severe side effects, and because he refused the H1N1 vaccine due to its toxicity.

I have been with my family physician since I was 22 years old. In over 30 years he has never overbooked appointments, and he spends time with me in discussion, truly listening. He has never over-prescribed or used pharmaceuticals to rush me out of the examination room. He has been respectful of my interest in alternative medicine, and during my first experience with cancer, went so far as to mail me an article on Native healing. Fabulous doctors abound. If you have one who will "fire" you for your opinions, run Forrest, run.

Remember: nothing is written in stone in the land of cancer. You can find thousands of stories of "unexplained" spontaneous remissions, healings and longevity of stage IV cancers and with what is currently considered terminal cancer. Almost none of these are being studied by the medical industry for commonalities and if a patient comes in with an explanation for the remission, it is considered anecdotal and is typically dismissed as such.

If you are given an "incurable" prognosis, *it is only incurable based on conventional methods and your particular practitioner's knowledge.* Do not accept another human's prediction of your life span. Cancer need not be a sentence, and can actually lead to a new beginning.

Remember… where there is life, there is always hope.

Question everything.

Highly inspiring:
TEDxSydney | False Hope? There's No Such Thing
Dr. Charlie Teo, Neurosurgeon
http://tinyurl.com/mug8trb

5

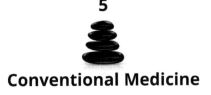

Conventional Medicine

"In all affairs it's a healthy thing now and then to hang a question mark on the things you have long taken for granted."
—Bertrand Russell

The standard recommendations for cancer in traditional medicine are surgery, radiation, and chemotherapy, depending on the stage and location of the cancer. Various drug regimens may be recommended as well. In the realm of allopathic (standard) medicine, doctors do not have the freedom to offer anything more than these protocols. Even if your doctor studies the research on trailblazing therapies outside of mainstream medicine or reads about the curative power of nutrition and finds the information convincing and legitimate, he/she is unable to recommend them or he/she risks peer ridicule, being reported, and further to that, a potential suspension.

I used traditional medicine for both of my cancer diagnoses and the following information is not designed to overwhelm or dissuade you. I share my experiences and research to help you make informed decisions that feel right for *you*—and to reduce your suffering.

You may require a barrage of tests from MRIs, PET scans and CT scans, x-rays, mammograms, ultrasound, and blood work, to biopsies.

The first time I was diagnosed, I had a surgical biopsy and was put under anesthetic at a hospital. The second time I had a needle biopsy at a clinic. Some women are not bothered by the procedure, but I found the needle biopsy barbaric and traumatic. Although doctors will refute it, from a common sense standpoint, firing a high-pressure gun-like needle into a tumor indicates the possibility of shattering it and spreading microscopic cancer cells. (Seeding of tumor cells following breast biopsy: a literature review[1].)

I had a lumpectomy both times (in 2010 it was called a partial mastec-

---

1   http://www.ncbi.nlm.nih.gov/pmc/articles/PMC3473763/

tomy) and in 1990 the lymph node resection required a deep cut into the armpit area. Numerous nodes were taken to determine if the cancer had spread. I have numbness in my arm from nerve damage, but fortunately did not suffer from lymphedema, which I attribute to the complementary treatments I underwent that were prescribed to offset the effects of conventional treatment.

In 2010 I opted out of the recommended lymph node resection. For breast cancer, this is standard procedure to determine if you have any metastatic activity. Understandably, most people want this information.

In my case, I did not want to further compromise my immune system because I had already lost numerous lymph nodes the first time. The lymphatic system is an important part of immunity and is the body's filtration for toxins. Removing nodes can cause lymphedema, a blockage of flow of the lymphatic fluid, which sometimes causes long-term swelling of the arm and hand, and less than optimal immunity. Also, if errant cancer cells had been found in my lymph nodes, the only recommendation in conventional medicine would have been chemotherapy.

Surgery

In Canada you will be assigned a surgeon, normally with expertise for your type of cancer. I researched surgeons and chose my own. Both times I sought surgeons known for breast conservation (saving as much of the breast as possible) with excellent reputations for both their skills and experience with breast cancer, and the surgeon's ability to communicate effectively and compassionately.

In the USA, be sure you fully understand costs and accreditation. Check with your health plan to learn exactly what is covered and what is not.

As previously mentioned, I highly recommend a composed and unbiased family member or friend to accompany you for note-taking, communication with others—basic project management. (I have created a free, downloadable planner that includes the following questions called, *My Wellness & Self-Care Planner*. Please see the back page of the book for the link.)

I have included an extensive list of questions for the doctors you may meet with. There might be things listed here that you are unconcerned about or do not feel you need to know, however, answers to these questions will help determine the course of treatment and better prepare you. *They are suggestions only.*

Questions for the surgeon:

- Why are you recommending this procedure?
- What are my options?
- Please explain exactly what is done in this type of surgery, before, during, and after.
- Has this type of surgery changed in the past twenty years or are you using advanced techniques?
- Is this your area of expertise?
- Will I have nerve damage?
- Will I have restricted mobility?
- What is the recovery time?
- What type of anesthesia will be administered?
- How long will I stay in the hospital?
- Are other organs affected?
- What exactly are all the potential risks and complications?
- What exactly are all the potential long-term side effects or conditions?
- What is required for follow-up care?

For breast cancer:

- If lymph node removal is recommended: How many nodes do you take and what is done to reduce the risk of lymphedema?
- Removing lymph nodes suppresses immune function. How will I improve my immunity after this surgery?
- How much breast tissue is being removed?
- What type of changes will I notice in my breast(s)?
- Will I need reconstruction?
- Will you take care with the aesthetics and breast conservation?
- Will you be leaving a titanium marker inside my breast? (These are used to identify the precise location of your tumor site.)
- Will a radiologist be inserting a wire localization in my breast pre-surgery and if so, please explain (these are placed to direct the surgeon).

If a mastectomy is recommended, do your research. Exactly why is this being recommended and does it truly increase your odds? Consider the emotional implications before rushing into a radical mastectomy.

If you do not understand what the surgeon has said, say so. Ask questions until you fully comprehend everything. Ask for written instructions if necessary.

The pathology report from the surgeon will label the stage of the cancer based on whether or not the tissue margins show that the cancer has spread to other areas and is also determined on the primary tumor's location and size. As difficult as it may be, try not to fixate on the stage. Many people are alive and well after stage IV diagnosis.

Radiation Oncologists

There are radiation oncologists and chemotherapy oncologists. The type and stage of your cancer pathology will determine which is recommended. These doctors are under strict guidelines and only their standard protocol is prescribed. They do not typically offer integrative (whole body/lifestyle) medicine.

Do not be afraid to ask a lot of questions. The role of an oncologist is in part to answer questions and address your concerns.

Questions for the radiation oncologist:

- Does radiation kill the cancer stem cells (the seeds, so to speak)?
- What are *all* of the adverse side effects and collateral damage to the healthy cells, bones, and organs of the body with this type of radiation?
- What is the irreversible damage (including nerve damage) that could occur to my body?
- Could there be hardening or scarring of tissue?
- Does this affect hair growth in the area (if applicable)?
- How will this affect the quality of my life?
- Will radiation affect my digestive system?
- How will this treatment affect my immune system?
- What are the statistical odds that I actually need radiation for my type of cancer?
- How are we planning on rebuilding my immune system due to any impairment from radiation?
- How do you determine the radiation protocol that is right for me?
- How long has this particular protocol been in use?
- Can you offer anything more advanced and cutting edge with lesser side effects?

- Radiation causes cancer, so why do we use radiation to destroy cancer and what are the chances of getting subsequent cancers from radiation therapy?
- I would like your honest answer to this question doctor. Would you take this protocol if you were diagnosed and would you recommend it to your family?

If you opt for radiation, you will have an appointment with the oncologist in a simulation room where the detailed planning is done. You may need to have a mask or mold created before the simulation.

Brachytherapy might be recommended, which is internal radiation placed inside the body or near the tumor site.

In the simulation room for external beam radiation, you will be placed in position and programming will be set to determine the delivery of the radiation dosage to a well-defined target volume and area. Simply put, a 360° image is taken via CT and this will give the oncologist information on where to target and how to best avoid collateral damage to surrounding organs.

Reference markers are attached on the skin. You may also require permanent dot-like tattoos. These are used to align your body to the beams at the precise placement each time.

Your schedule will be set for treatments. If you can, bring a friend or family member with you. The first time (1990) my treatment was five weeks long, so I went alone most of the time. The second time my treatment was for a much shorter period and I asked my sister to go with me. It eased my fear of the process and I appreciated the moral support. You will normally meet once a week with your oncologist during longer treatments.

You do not feel pain during the radiation; however, your skin might burn from the treatments. You may also feel heat inside of your body near the area that has been radiated (I did). Creams are recommended for burns. Ask if you can use organic calendula cream and aloe vera gel. These natural products do not contain harmful parabens. You could also purchase an aloe vera plant, break off small pieces, and apply the fresh aloe nectar directly to your skin to reduce burning and discoloration.

Radiation frequently causes fatigue and, depending on the location, can cause nausea. Listen to your body. It is working hard to repair the damage done to millions of healthy cells. Rest and sleep when you need it, no matter the time of day.

Keep eating! You may not feel hungry during treatment, but you need good nutrition to rebuild your body and recover properly.

Physiotherapy may be recommended later on. Follow the suggestions to prevent a restricted range of motion and potential lack of flexibility caused by surgery and/or radiation.

The most heart-wrenching part of radiation for both my sister and I was to pass the walking wounded and especially to see vulnerable children hooked up to chemo tubes and monitors. The energy of a cancer ward is not exactly healing. I have suggestions in subsequent chapters to help you maintain your emotional equilibrium.

When radiation is completed and your skin is healing, you may wish to take Himalayan sea salt and (non-ammonia) baking soda baths.

After surgery and radiation, a systemic skin disorder that I have (granuloma annulare) went feral. I suspect it was a combination of the effect of both therapies on my immune system and the psychological stress of a second cancer. After radiation I had a series of throat, ear, and sinus infections—over six months—which was clearly immune distress. I also went into menopause immediately after radiation, and experienced many unpleasant symptoms.

As a side note, I no longer have armpit hair since radiation. It could be considered a weird benefit, but it does illustrate the power of radiotherapy to permanently destroy healthy cells.

Weigh everything before making your decision if radiation is recommended.

Chemotherapy Oncologists
I researched chemotherapy ahead of my surgery, but was not given the recommendation for it. I have friends who have been prescribed a chemo regime and have had experience observing their journeys.

Questions for the chemotherapy oncologist:

- Does the chemotherapy kill the cancer stem cells (the seeds, so to speak)?
- What are *all* of the adverse side effects and collateral damage to the healthy cells, bone marrow, and organs of the body?
- What irreversible damage could occur to my body?
- How will this affect the quality of my life?

- How does chemotherapy affect my digestive system?
- How will this treatment affect my immune system?
- How are we planning on rebuilding my immune system due to the destruction of it through chemotherapy?
- What is 'chemo brain' and how long do the effects last?
- Will I lose all of my hair?
- How do you determine the type of chemotherapy that is right for me?
- What other drugs will be needed to offset the side effects of chemotherapy and exactly how much will they cost?
- (For intravenous chemo) Why do chemo nurses wear gloves and protective clothing and why is it considered a hazardous drug for nurses?
- What are the chances that this will completely cure me of cancer?
- What is the known mortality rate from using this treatment rather than from the actual cancer?
- How toxic is this drug, is it a known carcinogen, and can it cause secondary cancers?
- Is the goal with chemo a cured, healthy life or an extension of life?
- I would like your honest answer to this question doctor. Would you take this protocol if you were diagnosed and would you recommend it to your family?

Before considering chemotherapy, please make a truly informed decision. If you have reservations, ask to visit the chemo room to be given a tour of what is done in the procedure. Research the history of chemotherapy and the effects it will have on your quality of life, your body, and your mortality. Be sure to find out if the drug being prescribed is a known carcinogen.

Make sure you fully understand the math on the odds you are given in regards to the efficacy of the treatments. Sit on the recommendation in quiet contemplation to decide if it makes sense for you.

A family member who'd had a mastectomy was told her odds of reoccurrence would be reduced by 30% with chemotherapy. In a separate conversation with her oncologist, when she pressed, she was told the odds of reoccurrence after the mastectomy was approximately 16% without it.

So in doing the math, reducing 16% by 30% leaves 11.2%. In fact, you are actually only reducing your 16% odds by 5% (4.8%). I suspect when most people are told 30% they base it on 100%, and do not factor in the 16%. My family member decided she did not want to deal with the complications and collateral damage for the lowly 4.8% potential benefit. (She opted for a high nutrition regime, exercises religiously, and goes for emotional therapy when needed. The doctors had recommended a double mastectomy, which would have meant removing a healthy breast. She had only the affected breast removed followed by reconstruction. She also chose not to have radiation. She has had no recurrence in 19 years, has been in perfect health, and looks 10 years younger than her age.)

> *Actual calculations:*
> *16% chance of recurrence without chemotherapy.*
> *Reduce risk of recurrence by 30% if you take chemotherapy.*
> *Improvement = 16 x .30 = 4.8*
> *With chemo your chance of recurrence is now 16 − 4.8 = 11.2%.*
> *Without chemo your chance of recurrence was 16%.*
> *You only reduced your chances of recurrence by 16% − 11.2% = 4.8%*
> *Chemo provided a potential 4.8% improvement on the odds.*

In Canada, the statistical data oncologists use commonly comes from hands-on historic experience with patients. In my research, I found that in the USA most statistics used are based on S.E.E.R.: Surveillance Epidemiology and End Results[1]. These statistics are from approximately 28% of the population of the USA, and my understanding is that the stats are only based on three things:

1. Type of cancer
2. Date of diagnosis
3. Date of death

To reiterate, there is a lot of grey area in statistics. They do not include what type of complementary treatments were used, the diet and supplementation of the patient, the type of psychological support, stress levels pre-diagnosis, did the patient exercise, financial stresses because of cancer, marital issues, drug or alcohol abuse, etc. Also, there are numerous folks who have opted out of the conventional system and are healing via alternative methods, therefore are not included in the studies.

---

1   http://seer.cancer.gov/

If your instincts are telling you this treatment is not for you, listen. Please do not make decisions based on terror, pressure from *anyone*, or the collective beliefs based on propaganda.

For women with estrogen-positive breast cancer, I recommend researching Tamoxifen before agreeing to take it. It is designed to block all estrogen and will bring on sudden menopause. Review the toxicity and serious (and sometimes fatal) side effects of Tamoxifen before making a decision. It is considered a Group 1 carcinogenic (meaning it is a known carcinogenic with the highest rating of carcinogens) by the World Health Organization (1996) and the American Cancer Society.

List of carcinogens, American Cancer Society (Tamoxifen is in Group 1 and "Known to be human carcinogens"):

http://www.cancer.org/cancer/cancercauses/
othercarcinogens/generalinformationaboutcarcinogens/
known-and-probable-human-carcinogens

If you are an American, I recommend reading these two posts before making a decision on chemotherapy:

http://www.kevinmd.com/blog/2012/07/
oncologists-incentive-prescribe-expensive-treatments.html

http://www.healthbeatblog.com/
2009/01/a-very-open-letter-from-an-oncologist/

Video of importance:
TEDxLiverpool | How to make diseases disappear
Rangan Chatterjee
http://tinyurl.com/jfkjubl

6

Integrative and Complementary Medicine

*"A healer's power stems not from any special ability, but from maintaining the
courage and awareness to embody and express the universal healing power
that every human being naturally possesses."*
—Eric Micha'el Leventhal

An association exists in the province in which I live whose sole purpose
is to ensure that anyone diagnosed with cancer receives the proper care
and is aware of the required appointments. They make follow-up calls to
confirm that no one is missed within the busy system.

I spoke with a kind nurse from this organization and she asked if I had
any questions about the cancer process. I was planning my pre-surgery
trip to Mexico and I asked her what she knew of patients using integrative and complementary medicine. Her response was chilling. She said
that, unfortunately, most people opt to use it only when conventional
means have failed: in the latter stages of cancer when they are in a state
of desperation. With this in mind, it's important to stress that the success
rate drastically drops at this point, therefore, unfair to conclude that there
is no value to holistic treatments.

Complementary does not equal quack. Many renowned MDs and scientific researchers participate in alternative and complementary therapies—
this means anything outside of the surgery/radiation/chemotherapy/drug
standard of care model. In a conversation with one of my doctors about
the limited conventional options, she openly admitted that the only thing
medicine has to offer is the, and I quote, "slash-burn-poison" practice, and
that this approach to cancer is sorely lacking.

The number one goal of integrative, complementary, and alternative
medicine is to boost the immune system in a variety of ways with myriad of
protocols and therapies that allow the body to heal itself, as it is designed to
do. Integrative cancer care is a whole body approach commonly combined
with traditional medicine.

Typically, we are only familiar with conventional treatments for cancer because that is where the research and funding lies and that is where the ad campaign dollars are spent. It can be scary to take the road less traveled and you could be up against strong opposition if you venture off the path. There may be social, peer, medical, and familial pressure to follow the prescribed, standard protocols.

Nonetheless, waiting to use complementary medicine, nutrition, and natural remedies that boost your compromised immunity and help you heal as a last resort is like saying to a mechanic, "I'll fix the one flat tire and see how it goes," when you actually have three flat tires. Conventional medicine cannot offer you all of what your body requires for a genuine clean bill of health. Consider using complementary medicine *before* your body is depleted.

We can hand our bodies over to doctors—carte blanche—or we can take responsibility for our health by orchestrating our own healing plan and covering all aspects of wellbeing.

Why does cancer return if a patient has surgically removed tumors and has had radiation and/or chemotherapy? Most often because the body was not treated holistically to cure the root causes of what allowed cancer to flourish. Further to that, the treatments can cause cancer. Thousands of doctors and practitioners believe in the various pillars of health and in treating the whole body when we are in disease crisis. Any honest oncologist will agree that there is a negative impact on one's immune system when undergoing surgery, radiation, and especially chemotherapy.

Both times I went through my cancer journey I used both conventional medicine and alternative/complementary treatments. For the most part, I physically sailed through radiation treatments, which I attribute to the backup support I got alternatively. I never lost my appetite and, in fact, craved protein and ate hearty meals throughout. Both times I did not have any issues with radiation dermatitis (skin burning and blistering), but I did suffer fatigue.

Accredited naturopathic and homeopathic doctors, nutritionists, and acupuncturists who specialize in cancer handle areas that traditional doctors do not. They are usually well educated on the effects of radiation and chemotherapy and know what type of supplements, herbs, and remedies will assist in clearing the body of the negative effects of these potent and toxic treatments. A good practitioner also knows what adjunctive therapies can and cannot be taken during conventional treatments.

If, or when, your doctor tells you alternative treatments are 'hooey' or that good nutrition doesn't matter, I would like to offer you information on the terms of cancer research that you may not be aware of.

If something natural cures a certain type of cancer or aids in reducing tumors, you will never hear about it in a traditional medical institution. Understandably, doctors work with protocols that are scientifically and clinically tested and approved. However, cancer research is controlled and funded by the pharmaceutical industry. Clinical trials cost a lot (the average cancer drug costs $60-90 million to research). There are mainstream researchers seeking treatments that are well targeted and less brutal and damaging to the body, but again, under strict parameters that are bureaucratically governed.

When an up-and-coming researcher has discovered a natural cure, it will not go to clinical trial via traditional routes. Why not, you ask? If we are able to cure a disease so rampant and destructive, why on earth would a promising protocol or cancer cure go untested? For the simple reason that if it is not patentable and profitable—which natural cures are not—it never goes to trial. In fact, many natural cancer treatments have been silenced and fiercely discounted by the pharmaceutical industry and physicians and researchers have been scrutinized, even criminally charged, for uncovering natural cures.

The multi-billions raised in pink ribbon campaigns and cancer fundraisers do not go toward anything non-Pharma. Your doctor is aware of this and if you call mainstream cancer fundraising organizations, you will discover that even if a natural cure is showing promise in a lab somewhere, it will not be funded through their coffers unless it is patentable. The pharmaceutical industry is, for the most part, focused on treating and not preventing or curing cancer and it is ever seeking "blockbusters"—drugs that break the $1 billion mark, the tipping point where mega profits kick in. And the cost of these drugs has drastically escalated as the demand increases, in the same way profiteers jack up costs for basic necessities after a natural disaster.

Post-graduation, the subsequent education of oncologists is often sponsored by the pharmaceutical industry, which has no vested interest in teaching doctors about the latest findings in natural medicine or in the power of proper nutrition.

There have been countless documented cases of natural remedies and protocols that have aided and abetted in cancer cures and reduction and in "spontaneous remissions." If a simple raspberry, a mushroom, or the bark of a rainforest tree cures *anything*, the rigorous testing must be funded privately—and as outlined above, is no cheap feat.

Unfortunately greed prevents the world from knowing of these wonders—so far. When you can charge $1800 for a single pill to *offset* the effects of each chemotherapy treatment (my friend paid this for each of her 6 pills), it is of no benefit to the stockholders of Big Pharma to study the natural. The 'war on cancer' is a gargantuan, highly profitable business. Make no mistake—prevention and curing cancer is not lucrative. Period.[1]

The idea of awarding cancer its elevated campaign status, with special combat zone terminology and politically restricted and regulated research, began in the passing of the National Cancer Act in 1971, instigated by the 'illustrious' Richard Nixon. The concept was the impetus of two high-pressure lobbyists. Prior to that, the renegade scientists who populated the landscape of cancer research had the freedom to chase whatever hypotheses they had conjured.

Since then, the lexicon of the 'war on cancer' has spread and infiltrated our collective consciousness like a virus. But if we stop and look at the hard facts, the war has been lost. The goal of the lobbyists was to gain notoriety through eradicating cancer by America's 200th birthday. Instead, cancer has escalated exponentially to a one-in-three epidemic. Too many of the victories in survivorship have been pyrrhic; they inflict such a devastating toll on the victor that the triumph is questionable.

When anything fails as epically as has the rigid methodology for cancer, all logic dictates that revision and reinvention are in order. The time has come for medicine to abide by the Hippocratic Oath that doctors swear to: avoid overtreatment, prevent disease, and in essence, *do no harm*. After almost five decades, a 'truce on cancer' is long overdue.

The pathology of cancer is not a single disease, but many multi-faceted diseases that require highly individualized treatments. We now have such precise testing that over-diagnosis is an area being monitored by the medical field. Abnormalities are reported back to the patient and minor cancers are over-treated—cancers that would never have shown symptoms or harmed the patient had they not known. As an example, pap tests have been changed to a three-year period instead of one year for precisely this

---

1   http://www.fool.com/investing/general/2015/03/28/5-freakishly-expensive-cancer-drugs.aspx

reason. The cervix has cycles of cell change and abnormalities that can heal without intervention.

Too frequent testing can result in false positive results and cause undue anxiety and unnecessary treatment.

An organization called Codex Alimentarius[1] (meaning food code) was designed to focus on food safety, but is using its power to promote worldwide restrictions on information and distribution of vitamins, herbs, and supplements. Codex standards are enforceable through the World Trade Organization.

You must be extremely discerning when you do your own research to find the right practitioners and optimal therapies. In any field you will find the good, the bad, and the ugly. Check the reputation of anyone you work with both in traditional and alternative settings, and get referrals. Use common sense and gut instinct to make decisions—not fear, desperation, and/or panic.

A friend of mine spent a small fortune at a greed-based treatment clinic for a chronic condition. I, on the other hand, went to a humble clinic in Puerto Vallarta. Dr. Jose Luis Romo is an MD who has traveled the world looking for treatments and cures for cancer and, for the past two decades, has dedicated himself to the study of holistic healing. I saw him on the recommendation of a friend who had attended his clinic many years for preventative treatments. I was given intravenous chelation with vitamin C, ozone IV therapy, colonic hydrotherapy, Papimi treatments, and nutritional detox along with the Budwig protocol. I took various botanicals and supplements. Costs were clearly outlined and reasonable.

While undergoing surgery and radiation in Canada, I went to a Body Talk practitioner. After treatment, I returned to Mexico and was under the care of an intuitive acupuncturist/herbalist. We gently rebooted my immune system. I used the balance of my life savings for these various treatments, but they were affordably priced and administered by compassionate and caring people. Also, I was in a place I adore, surrounded by nature, beauty, and sunshine.

Should you choose to solely go the alternative route, do it with commitment and preparedness. Do extensive research and chart a solid wellness plan under the care and guidance of an expert with successful

---

1   http://www.natural-health-information-centre.com/codex-alimentarius.html

and proven cancer protocols. Be sure you are dealing with the emotional and spiritual aspects of illness with professional support or you may find yourself adrift.

A plethora of gentle complementary therapies exist which are effective for cancer. Many of these can be used in conjunction with traditional medicine or post treatment to reboot and rebuild the immune system. A personalized regime can be integrated. Below is a list of prevalent therapies being used worldwide.

Areas of Integrative/Complementary/Alternative Therapies to Consider

- Naturopathic oncology doctor
- Gerson therapy
- Chelation therapy (removes toxic metals)
- Hyperbaric oxygen therapy
- Ozone intravenous therapy (antioxidant, oxygenates cells, detoxifies, helps body absorb nutrients)
- High dose vitamin C intravenous therapy
- Alpha lipoic acid (ALA) intravenous therapy
- Curcumin intravenous therapy (water soluble type)
- Myers' Cocktail intravenous therapy (magnesium chloride, calcium, B vitamins, and Vitamin C: interestingly Wikipedia called it a modern day "snake oil." This shows how the industry is seeding misinformation; basic minerals and vitamins cannot be considered "snake oil." Anyone can edit Wikipedia so please do not get your information there. I personally edited out the snake oil reference due to its blatant inaccuracy.)
- Breast cancer: Cryoablation (freezing of the tumor)[1]
- Chinese medicine and acupuncture
- Reiki and energy balancing
- Biodynamic craniosacral therapy
- Trauma therapy
- Ayurveda (Hindu traditional medicine)
- Biological dentistry (For the removal of mercury amalgam fillings. After researching, I removed all amalgam fillings in 1990 to mitigate mercury toxicity)
- Chiropractic

---

1 http://icecure-medical.com/

- Gentle detox of gut, liver, and urinary tract
- Heavy metal detoxification (heavy metal toxicity is more common that we realize and has a negative effect on health and impedes healing)
- Naturopathic testing for candida or fungal overgrowth
- Hyperthermia treatments
- Light therapy
- Infrared sauna
- Homeopathy
- Virotherapy vaccines (Rigvir® non-toxic and specific to types of cancer)
- PEMF magnetic field therapy (especially brain cancer)
- Colonics and coffee enemas
- Sound and Rife GB4000 Frequency Therapy[1]
- Also: Shattering Cancer with Resonant Frequencies (important work)[2]
- Parasite cleanse (parasites greatly suppress the immune system)
- Proper hydration with purified water
- Body Talk[3]
- Alternative to mammography: thermography detection

Botanical Medicines

Thousands of natural medicines are used to treat cancer around the world. I have done extensive research and have carefully filtered the list to comprise of the "heavy-hitters" that have demonstrated curative success with cancer, enhance immunity, and diminish or eliminate symptoms. A combination of botanicals chosen with a qualified practitioner along with a high nutrition diet is a powerful restoration plan.

- Medical cannabis oil: Amazing results have been recorded from this powerful medicine.
- B-17: Laetrile, derived from apricot pits, allegedly more effective with hyperthermia.
- Curcumin: Found in turmeric, is a powerhouse for inhibiting cancer cell mutation and metastasis. It is an anti-inflammatory and can actually

---

1 https://www.theguardian.com/science/2015/oct/31/ ultrasound-cancer-research-hifu-bone-trial
2 https://youtu.be/1w0_kazbb_U
3 http://vibranttransformation.com/healingbodymind/

kill various types of cancer. You can find many studies on curcumin. Choose high absorption, quality brands. Some studies say it is protective against the harmful effects that occur as a result of radiotherapy, and that curcumin actually enhanced the effect of radiotherapy.

• Graviola/Guanabana/Soursop: The leaves, bark, and roots are considered nature's chemotherapy—without the side effects. This potent substance is anti-viral, anti-bacterial, anti-fungal, and anti-tumoral. I took a fresh tincture post-radiation for eight months, which was made by my acupuncturist from her own trees in Mexico. Get expert advice.

• CLA: Conjugated linoleic acid, studies have shown excellent results in reduction of tumors in certain cancers.

• Sea Buckthorn (not for use pre-surgery)

• Artemisia Annua/Sweet Wormwood/Qing Hao

• Pau D'Arco/Taheebo

• Cat's claw and burdock root: For the lymphatic system.

• Magnesium: Deficiency is rampant due to our soil's depletion of minerals. Get tested if possible.

• Lycopene: Studies show reduced risk in prostate and breast cancer.

• Krill Oil

• Spirulina

• Moringa

• Sulforaphane: Found in cruciferous vegetables and available in supplements.

• N-Acetyl-L-cysteine

• Glutathione

• Oldenlandia[1]

• Scutellaria barbata and scutellaria baicalensis[2]

• Essential oil therapy: Especially frankincense, myrrh, and sandalwood.

• Flower essences

• Green tea: Powerful healing catechins.

• Wheatgrass

• Chlorophyll

• Mistletoe/Iscador

---

1   http://www.itmonline.org/arts/oldenlandia.htm
2   https://www.mskcc.org/cancer-care/integrative-medicine/herbs/scutellaria-baicalensis

- Indole-3-carbinol: Improves outcome for estrogen-enhanced cancers including breast, endometrial, and cervical.
- Essiac tea
- Protocel
- Reishi Cordyceps: Medicinal mushrooms.
- Kelp: Iodine deficiency is common.
- Vitamin D: Get tested for deficiency, 20 minutes of sun daily is still the best source. Deficiency is common in cancer patients and is crucial to healing.
- Vilcacora Forte
- Sangre de Drago
- Micronutrients
- Tahuari
- Wobenzym: For inflammation.
- Neem
- Resveratrol
- Selenium
- Chromium
- Silica
- Raw cacao
- Aloe vera
- Probiotics and fermented products for gut health.
- High quality zeolites, activated charcoal, papain, and bee pollen detoxify and protect the body from harmful effects of radiation.

Integrative and Complementary Clinics
Cancer clinics in Canada and the USA are under highly restricted rules and regulations and that is why you will find different therapies offered elsewhere; however, there are many cancer treatment centers in North America offering excellent alternative therapies.

The following is a small sampling of successful integrative cancer clinics:

Dr. Jose Luis Romo MD
La Flor de la Salud, Puerto Vallarta and Puebla, Mexico
http://flordelasalud.com/en/
I was treated by Dr. Romo in 2010 for cancer at the Puerto Vallarta clinic and had excellent complementary and integrative care. Dr. Romo has

since opened Clinica Flor de la Salud in Puebla with accommodations and a holistic meal plan. Treatments include IV chelation, ozone, nutrition, colonic hydrotherapy, detoxification, Papimi treatment, emotional counseling, and more.

Dr. Janelle Murphy, ND
Calgary Integrative Medicine, Calgary, Canada
http://www.calgarymed.ca
Dr. Murphy's passion lies in treating cancer and chronic diseases through naturopathic avenues in an integrative approach. She has advanced clinical training and is a member of the Oncology Association of Naturopathic Physicians. She is certified in Naturopathic Oncology. Tamara Pynn, a Certified Holistic Nutritional Consultant, is also on staff at this progressive clinic and colonic hydrotherapy is available.

Dr. Eugene Quan ND
Western Naturopathic, Calgary, Canada
http://www.westernnaturopathic.com/
Dr. Quan has had a high success rate with late stage cancers by using stringent protocols starting with allergy and leaky gut testing, detoxification cleansing, dietary changes, hyperthermia, intravenous therapies and more.

Dr. D. Wittel MD, PhD, President, Chelation Therapy Medical Association
Chelation Medical Centers of the Okanagan,
Penticton and Kelowna, B.C., Canada
http://chelationbc.com
Dr. Wittel is an MD who practices holistic, scientifically valid medicine. He specializes in IV therapies of vitamin C, hydrogen peroxide, glutathione, Myers' Cocktail, and more.

Dr. Erwin Weijnen
Paracelsus Clinic for Biological Medicine, Nuremberg, Germany
http://www.paracelsus-praxisklinik.de/biologische-medizin/
krebserkrankungen/
Dr. Weijnen is an expert in all aspects of holistic biological medicine. The clinic offers nutritional counseling, hyperthermia, colonic hydrotherapy, craniosacral, ostheopathy, Dorn Preuss therapy, and herbal chemotherapeutic treatments: Artemisia annua and laetrile.

Dr. Elias Gutierrez, MD, Dr. Martha Garcia, MD,
Dr. Fernando Cruz, MD, Dr. Sergio Michel, MD
Bio-Medical Centre, Tijuana, Mexico
http://www.hoxseybiomedical.com
This renowned clinic, once called the Hoxsey Clinic, was moved from the USA to Mexico because it was under attack by the AMA for treating cancer. It is famous for the Hoxsey formula and uses a variety of alternative and conventional treatments with a long track record of success with cancer.

Dr. Antonio Jimenez, MD
Hope4Cancer Institute, Baja California, Mexico
http://www.hope4cancer.com/
Dr. Antonio Jimenez is the founder of the Hope4Cancer Institute in Mexico. He has used leading-edge non-toxic treatment options for even the most dire types and stages of cancer for the past 25 years. Available treatments include virotherapy, sono-photo dynamic therapy, hyperthermia, AARSOTA bio-immunotherapy, and IV protocols.

Dr. Patrick Vickers, DC
Northern Baja Gerson Center, Mexico
http://www.gersontreatment.com/
The Gerson Center offers a comprehensive, holistic, all-natural approach. The protocol has shown great success with cancer using stringent dietary therapy, hyperbaric oxygen, Coley's Toxins, enemas, dendritic cell therapy, biological dentistry, hyperthermia, and more.

Dr. Carlos M. Garcia, MD
The Utopia Wellness Clinic, Oldsmar, Florida, USA
http://utopiawellness.com/intensive-medical-program-for-cancer/
Dr. Garcia is a holistic physician using immunotherapy, psychological counseling, detoxification, lymphatic massage, diet, chelation, and oxygen therapy with an intensive personalized program designed to address the root causes of cancer.

Dr. Raymond Hilu, MD
Clinica Hilu, Marbella, Spain
http://www.clinicahilu.com/
Dr. Hilu is a medical maverick and has traveled the world to study new

technologies. He specializes in cellular medicine and was the only scientific collaborator trained by Dr. Johanna Budwig. His clinic uses cutting-edge diagnostics, detoxification, and an array of non-toxic therapies such as Papimi treatment, focused infrared, and orthomolecular protocols with a body, mind, spirit approach.

Dr. Manuela Malaguti-Boyle, PhDc, MHSc NMD, FIO
Cassia Clinic, Queensland, Australia
http://www.cliniciansolutions.com
Dr. Malaguti-Boyle actively embraces collaboration with conventional health professionals to best support the body's healing and help patients cope with the toxic side effects of traditional therapies. She is a Nutritional & Herbal Medicine Cancer Specialist and is certified in Integrative Oncology. Non-toxic therapies for immune stimulation include nutrition, chelation, detoxification, and psychological support.

Dr. Ron Hunninghake, MD, Dr. Nia Stephanopoulos-Chichura, MD,
Dr. Jennifer Mead, ND, Dr. Timothy Lawton, MD, Anne Zauderer, DC
Riordan Clinic Functional and Integrative Medicine, Kansas, USA
http://www.riordanclinic.org
The Riordan Clinic is a not-for-profit organization with a 40-year history of evaluating and lab testing, prolozone therapy, magnetic therapy, lymphatic drainage, ultraviolet blood irradiation, IV, and nutrition therapies. Their mission is to "stimulate an epidemic of health."

Dr. Stanislaw Burzynski MD
Burzynski Clinic, Houston, Texas, USA
http://www.burzynskiclinic.com/
This clinic was established in 1977 with a Hippocratic "first, do no harm" philosophy and a highly personalized approach based on genetic testing. Dr. Burzynski pioneered the use of biologically active peptides for the treatment of cancer and his clinic is internationally recognized. He has had noteworthy success with brain cancer patients.

Dr. Isai Castillo, MD
Dr. Castillo's Clinic, Tijuana, Mexico
http://www.drcastillo.com
Dr. Isai Castillo is an MD who blends complementary and traditional medi-

cine with a mission to give people the best of both worlds to obtain optimum health. His clinic offers detoxification and cleansing, immune building, IV treatments, and more. His work is targeted to all types of disease.

There are many more alternative centers worldwide doing amazing work to eradicate cancer; I cite these to give you a starting point. If you decide to go to a private clinic, ask for exact costs in writing and get referrals from patients. Do your homework and do not make complete payments in advance.

If it is financially feasible, a spouse, partner, or loved one may be open to joining you for preventative treatments at the clinic of your choice.

Cancer Coaching

An excellent way to work through your decision making process is to discuss your options with a qualified and unbiased cancer coach. I highly recommend a consultation in the event of a stage IV diagnosis.

Wellness Coach Valerie Warwick RN[1] was a chemotherapy nurse for 17 years and transitioned into Functional and Orthomolecular Medicine. She can explain the pros and cons of your choices with expertise and help you chart a plan.

In 2004, health and cancer coach Chris Wark[2] cured himself of stage III colon cancer without chemotherapy. He promotes taking control of your own health through diet and lifestyle transformation.

Alternative Testing

A pioneering blood test invented by Dr. Johannes Coy and Dr. Martin Grimm at the German Cancer Research Center at the University of Heidelberg, Germany is available for the early detection of cancer. This is a biomarker-based detection and characterization of carcinomas. These two doctors received a Nobel Prize in chemistry.

The General Hospital of the University of Tubingen offers the test for international and domestic patients. (The test is offered to German citizens once a year at no cost.)

In Canada, the chemotherapy currently administered is not tested for its effectiveness on each particular tumor or cancer, meaning it is not a personalized treatment. What may be effective for one person with the

---

1   http://www.mywellnesstutor.com
2   http://www.chrisbeatcancer.com/

same cancer may not be for the next. The "Greek Test," developed by RGCC—a genetic lab—involves the non-invasive capture of malignant cells and tests the cultures with all modern chemotherapy agents, a multitude of natural agents, and the genetic expression of the cancer. This critical information will tell you which therapy would work and which would be ineffective for your cancer pathology.

In British Columbia, Canada, Dr. Janessa Laskin, an oncologist and senior scientist, has had tremendous success with personalized onco-ge-nomics. This involves identifying the gene mutations that direct a patient's cancer. The team has the capacity to sequence (test) 6,000 cancers each year and has just received the promise of further provincial funding. Currently, only incurable cancer patients residing in B.C. are eligible.

Another privately funded Bio Tech company doing similar work—identifying cancer genes and biological markers of disease, prognosis, and drug response—is soon to launch in Canada.

ONCOblot[1]® is a non-invasive tissue of origin test and is FDA approved. This test reveals the origin of malignant cells on 25 types of cancer.

Toxicity

Unfortunately planet Earth has become a toxic place to live and toxins sit in our cells. They can block absorption of the nutrients we need to heal. It would be of great benefit to have a parasite cleanse and detoxify your intestinal tract, urinary tract, and your liver under the supervision of an experienced practitioner. The liver is of incredible importance because of the control it has on over 400 functions of the body. If it is congested in any way, it will impede health and healing.

At week two, when my doctor in Mexico recommended colonics, my reaction was less than tactful. I was already incensed with a second cancer, but an assault to my nether region? He laughed and explained the benefits and after much thought, I agreed to a round of three colonics at a clinic which housed a modern European system. Even though I was highly resistant, I felt euphoric afterward. By the third colon flush, I had the sensation of floating on air. I share this with you because I was the least likely person to get a colonic.

Our colons and livers are assaulted daily by toxins. In the healing process, the cleaner your system, the better. We humans can have many

1   http://oncoblotlabs.com/

pounds of toxic poo stagnating in our colons and it blocks the way for the absorption of much-needed nutrients, vitamins, and minerals. Some MDs will argue the benefits, but do some research for yourself.

Electromagnetic Pollution

We are subjected to an enormous amount of electromagnetic pollution and nobody yet knows (or admits to) the extent of the implications to our health. Parts of Europe are restricting the amount of electromagnetic usage, but in North America there is no limit. Receiving is not the biggest issue; the transmitting of signals is purported to have the most health dangers.

If you live near or under towers, you may wish to consider moving in the future. Because we cannot see it, taste it, or smell it, we do not consider it a risk. Taking into account that cancer is now a one-in-three proposition, I suspect we will learn in the future the real and profound damage being done to our systems. Our bodies are magnetic, so be assured there is an effect. Studies are being done and the World Health Organization has declared that cellphone radiation may be linked to brain cancer because of the interference with the body's internal electrical and electro-chemical signaling systems.

Some suggestions for reducing your exposure to electromagnetic energy are:

- Removing all computers, modems, and cellphones from your bedroom (keep your phone far away from you when you sleep—distance matters).
- Shutting off your modem at night to reduce the amount of exposure.
- Using ear buds (*not* a wired hands-free set) or speaker mode on long calls and limit usage of cellphones if possible.
- Texting more, talking less.
- Keeping your cellphone away from your body and never carrying it in pockets and especially bras. If you insist on carrying it near your body, put it on flight mode.
- Avoiding electric blankets. (Use old-fashioned hot water bottles if need be.)
- Avoiding microwaves. (Zapping your food with high-frequency radiation waves of heat has been studied and found to be harmful and changes the molecular structure of food.)
- Using cellphone, laptop, and tablet radiation shields. (Do research on efficacy before buying.)

Environmental Toxins

Toxins are now a part of everyday life unless you live in a remote area growing your own organic food. Chemical toxins may enter the cells of our tissue and interact with genetic material. We are constantly subjected to pesticides, fungicides, and herbicides and that is why it is a very good idea to gently detoxify. If you are subjected to obvious harsh toxins, chemicals, or mold, do your best to remove yourself from exposure to:

- Heavy metals
- Mold
- Chlorine
- An excess of medications
- Cigarette or cigar smoke
- Highly polluted areas with exhaust emissions
- Working with dangerous chemicals or gases
- Round Up (glyphosate)
- Aspartame (an excitotoxin with 92 known harmful side effects[1])
- MSG (excitotoxin)

Natural Skin Cancer Remedies

I include this section because, as I was writing this book, a mysterious mole appeared—and began to grow—behind my earlobe. I researched natural cures in the event that there were any suspicious cells present in the mole. I tried one remedy I had read about before booking a doctor appointment.

It was simply organic coconut oil and baking soda. I added the baking soda for a few days, but applied coconut oil every morning and night for less than two weeks. I also added frankincense oil, but only twice. It began to dry and harden. Lo and behold—it fell off without a trace! I am not suggesting you let suspicious lesions grow without having them checked by a professional, but you could research the following and test your choice pre-appointment.

- Organic virgin coconut oil and baking soda (non-aluminum)
- Red clover extract
- Eggplant extract
- Black raspberry seed oil

---

1   http://www.sweetpoison.com/aspartame-side-effects.html

- Myrrh oil
- Frankincense oil
- Iodine
- Citrus oil

An all-encompassing source of information on alternative therapies available around the world is the documentary series, *The Truth About Cancer*[1]. It can be overwhelming to watch, but has highly revealing and life-saving information. Ty Bollinger's quest is controversial, as is anything that challenges the status quo, but it is a critical body of material for anyone with a diagnosis or history of cancer.

Massimo Mazzucco's documentary, *Cancer: The Forbidden Cures*[2], is a must watch to understand how the medical system evolved into what it is today.

Vitamin & Supplement Tip
Remembering to take supplements as prescribed can be a challenge. Sometimes bottles in a cupboard remain forgotten—out of sight, out of mind. I have devised a system that is effective. I place all of my vitamins and supplements in a wicker tray in small bowls. The tray is neatly tucked away and in the morning I take it out and place the daily regime in a pretty ceramic bowl and keep it on the counter. If I am going out for the whole day, I take the vitamins in a to-go case. You can get day-of-the-week pill cases at the drugstore or dollar store.

Chemo Tips
I did not take chemotherapy but, after 50, I started to lose more hair. I discovered that biotin and L-Cysteine along with N-Acetyl-L-cysteine helps. Instead of a handful of hair to clean from the drain each shampoo, I now only lose a smattering. My hair is also growing faster. This combination may help with new hair growth after treatment.

A natural scalp mask that can be used for hair growth and conditioning is a combination of two parts castor oil and one part olive oil, slightly warmed. Castor oil is a natural wonder; it thickens, softens, and encourages hair growth. It can be used on eyebrows and eyelashes for growth as well. It is an effective skin moisturizer and can be mixed with almond oil or

---

1   https://go2.thetruthaboutcancer.com
2   http://topdocumentaryfilms.com/cancer-forbidden-cures/

coconut oil for a less sticky consistency. Once a scar has closed, it can reduce scar tissue if you have had surgery.

You may be aware of the bone broth craze. Our grandmothers, and the matriarchs before them, knew the power of simmered bone broth. The whole chicken-soup-when-you-are-sick has chops. It is excellent for gut health and has immune boosting properties. I make chicken bone broth infrequently, so I use a supplement daily in its place: hydrolyzed collagen (from pasture fed cows). It is a powder that dissolves in water and is tasteless. If you are vegetarian, you can take marine collagen. Since taking this supplement, my skin has become a bit firmer and smoother. Not only is it good for the gut but all collagen in your body: joints, hair, nails and skin. Gelatin can repair damage to the gut and improve digestion.[1]

If you have had chemotherapy, you may notice a difference in the texture of your skin. Bone broth and hydrolyzed collagen can help repair the damage.

Cancer treatments can wreak havoc on the digestive system and good gut health is imperative for overall wellness. Consider a high quality probiotic to maintain good bacteria in your digestive tract, especially if you are taking prescription drugs or chemotherapy.

Skin Care Tips

Many of the lotions on store shelves are toxic and, regrettably, found to be carcinogenic.

I have used commercially prepared skin products for years, but in my research I learned that the skin absorbs a high percentage of what we rub on it, thus absorbing the toxins in the product which then swim through our blood stream and infiltrate our organs. A 60-70% absorption rate caught my attention. Slathering myself daily in toxic creams and lotions was not something I wanted to continue doing.

I still use commercially manufactured foundation on my face and have not completely switched my make-up (due to cost), but I now use natural, handmade lotions for my body. I apply coconut oil with natural lotion as a facial moisturizer. I use natural, locally made soap from the health food store; it costs $1.29 a bar from the bulk soap stand.

Because of wicked hot flashes it took me a long time to switch to natural deodorant, but I have done so to stop subjecting my lymph nodes

---

1   http://wellnessmama.com/7419/gelatin-uses/

to aluminum compounds and other noxious chemicals and preservatives.

I make a body scrub that makes my skin soft and smooth with only two ingredients: organic cold-pressed coconut oil and white sugar. Mix it to a consistency that is grainy for a good shower scrub. I also gently apply it to my face.

I am not a soaking-in-a-hot-bath kind of person, but if you are, I highly recommend you make your own bath soaks or buy holistic versions; many standard bath products are toxic.

Try to avoid all parabens: Benzyl Paraben, Methyl Paraben, N-Prophyl Paraben, N-Butyl Paraben, Ethyl Paraben, Isobutyl Paraben. These preservatives are found in most

cosmetics and creams and are linked to breast cancer.

Check this infographics chart on 12 toxic ingredients to avoid in cosmetics and skin care products[1].

1 http://www.mindbodygreen.com/0-5971/12-Toxic-Ingredients-to-AVOID-in-Cosmetics-Skin-Care-Products-Infographic.html

7

It *Is* All About You Right Now

"For those of you who struggle with guilt regarding self-care, answer this question: What greater gift can you give to those you love than your own wholeness?"
—Shannon Tanner

If you have ever flown, you have heard the flight attendants give instructions in the case of an emergency. They always tell you to first put on your own oxygen mask before your child's. That is because if you pass out, you cannot help your child, or anyone.

The same goes for cancer. You come first. This is not about what is best for your husband, mother, wife, child, boss—or anybody else. This is a time for what is absolutely best for you. If you do not take care of yourself properly, you run the risk of not being around for others anyway.

I overheard a hunched and fatigued-looking woman speaking to a social worker at the hospital. She said she was from a culture where the mother is considered the maid and sole organizer of the home. She had gone through radiation and was undergoing chemotherapy and was extremely ill, yet her husband and teenage daughters still expected her to keep up with all of her previous duties in the same way as before the cancer diagnosis and they refused to help. I was concerned for her survival based on the lack of compassion and care she was being shown and by how run-down she appeared.

If you have been the chief cook, bottle washer, and chauffeur, it is time for others to step up and not only take care of themselves, but take care of you. If you are a single mom or dad and have small children, there is likely someone in your world who can assist you at this time. If your spouse has not participated much before, now is the time.

Guilt seems to play a huge role in the decisions people make during their journey to wellness. But guilt and people-pleasing are inappropriate for healing. When we have forsaken our own needs for others, we become irritable and resentful of those we are in service to.

Ask yourself what you need right now. If you want a trip away from everyone, express it and find a way to make it happen. If you adore fresh tulips or the taste of premium honeybush tea, indulge. If you need solitude, ask for it. If your body is begging for sleep and rest, take it. Make yourself as comfortable as possible right now and learn to say no.

I have a friend who went away and for six months, slept 12 hours a day. Her new friends teased her about it, but she was non-apologetic. Her body was screaming for sleep. She did not argue with it and she did not feel guilty for it. She is fortunate to have the type of business that allows her to work remotely, but the point is, she gave herself permission to rest and recalibrate her system—minus all guilt.

You need to allow yourself the best tender loving care right now. Minimize your stress as much as is humanly possible. Let go of preconceived notions about your role(s) and set clear boundaries. Don't assume others will intuit your wishes. Sit down with your family and explain your requirements clearly if need be.

I am a crazy list writer and one thing I discovered during cancer was that lists will wait. The world continues to turn even when these "important" things are put on hold.

I also learned that I have a strong sense of self-preservation. That means saying no to demands that I think will exhaust me or to things I will detest. In the '90s (après cancer) when I told an out-of-province manager that I would be shutting my fax machine off until 8 a.m. each day, he was irate. He wanted the freedom to send me corporate missives at all hours. My office was next to my bedroom and if you have ever heard a fax ring, you know it is loud and screeching. I let him know that if he needed to fax me at all hours, he would have to pay for a separate office. I stood firm. Sleep is important to health and I was tired of having it disrupted inappropriately for someone else's convenience.

Another thing to bear in mind is that your life is valuable and putting the future financial comforts for your family ahead of your healing just doesn't make sense. Of course, you do not want to saddle your family with bankruptcy, but if there are reserves such as family savings, equity in a mortgage, a line of credit, etc. then use them. If your heart tells you to go elsewhere for treatments or recovery, listen. Money can show up from the strangest places and things will come together when you decide to choose what you know is right. If you were to ask your family if they would prefer "stuff" over having you live longer, I think you know what the answer would be.

Do not martyr yourself. You are loved and cherished by those around you. I beseech you to make *you* number one right now as a part of your wellness plan. Your life may depend on it.

Relax
Rejuvenate
Refresh
Restore
Revive
Reboot
Reinvent

Here is a playlist for restful slumbering:
Lynne's Sleep Meditations
https://tinyurl.com/mebss8x

8

Make an Integrative Wellness and Self-Care Plan

"Each patient carries his own doctor inside him."
—Norman Cousins
Anatomy of an Illness

If you carry on doing whatever you were doing before you were diagnosed, you are not addressing the imbalances in your body and life.

Cancer is a "whole person" disease and it is unlikely that your doctors will have a holistic plan for you. Currently, their job is to solely address their area of expertise. In order to build a robust immune system, you need an integrative wellness plan to bring you to homeostasis; equilibrium in the body with a return to stabilized health.

It is unrealistic to expect a person who is newly diagnosed to make a sweeping lifestyle transformation all at once. However, change can begin with a Kaizen (continuous change for the better) approach; start now with the easiest first. The number of things to avoid and consider modifying can be overwhelming, but making shifts in increments can make a big difference.

Also, you cannot effectively do this alone. Having a trustworthy healing professional with experience in cancer to guide and support you is the best way to navigate. Because I sought them, I found a team of wonderful wise women (and one good man) who were dedicated to helping me heal with a wholehearted generosity; a collective effort and love that still awes me.

The following is a list of suggestions for your wellness plan. Some ideas will resonate strongly, others will not. One size does not fit all; listen to your inner guidance system on what feels best as a customized plan and start with what is simplest to implement. Fear based changes defeat the goal of wellness. Do things that inspire you to take your self-care to a new level—one that you have always deserved.

Feel free to download and print your free PDF of *My Wellness & Self-Care Planner* addendum and place it in a binder. You can journal and track appointments with this guidebook as well. See the link in the back page of this book.

Remember to include the physical, emotional, psychological, spiritual, nutritional, environmental, and social, with a review of your work life for a holistic, whole-life approach to healing.

This list of ideas includes activities that are generic as well as specific to men or women:

- Evaluating recommended traditional protocols
- Researching complementary and alternative treatments
- Undertaking detoxification with a qualified practitioner
- Engaging in a high-quality nutrition plan
- Sourcing and taking immune boosting supplements/botanicals
- Outsourcing chores/work
- Walking (hand-in-hand with a loved one—even better)
- Swimming
- Fishing
- Dancing
- Playing pool
- Accessing infrared saunas
- Participating in meditation
- Reaping the benefits of visualization
- Learning about and practicing EFT Tapping
- Connecting with psychological and spiritual therapy or coaching
- Celebrating life by delectable picnicking with friends, anywhere
- Taking nature time-outs
- Singing
- Golfing
- Attending classical music and concerts
- Swinging in a hammock
- Joining drumming circles
- Writing in a gratitude journal
- Resting, napping, and sleeping sufficiently
- Reading (magazines and blogs are great if your attention span is short)
- Playing games
- Abstaining from checking your portfolio
- Coloring in themed, detailed coloring books
- Watching comedic movies

- Having a makeover (check for free programs available for cancer patients)
- Getting a hot shave
- Enjoying a man-pedicure/foot massage
- Driving through the countryside on back roads
- Drinking lots of water to cleanse and hydrate—important*
- Hanging out at libraries and interesting bookstores
- Taking a child to an animated kid's movie
- Visiting museums
- Using aromatherapy
- Attending yoga
- Exploring Tai Chi
- Learning about Qi Gong
- Doing breathing exercises
- Utilizing the power of prayer and ritual
- Enjoying a light massage
- Experiencing reflexology
- Indulging in Epsom salt and essential oil baths
- Painting as art therapy (Paint Nite[1] has relaxing art evenings in many cities and many cancer support centers have free painting classes)
- Meandering in botanical gardens and parks
- Borrowing a dog to take for a walk
- Taking weekend trips to the mountains, ocean, or a tranquil place
- Saying NO (No is a complete sentence.)

Please rest. Let go of any guilt that drives you to go-go-go. It is nobody's business how much you sleep, read, or rest. Relaxation and downtime is an incredibly important part of your recovery. It's healing.

Also, imbue your life with as much beauty as possible right now. You may be in clinical settings that are stark and sometimes soul sucking, so seek gorgeousness and that which soothes you; surround yourself with beauty and immerse yourself in wonder.

Most cancer survivors I have spoken with have never made a post-cancer healing plan. They race back to work and the status quo. Maybe because it was a second cancer, I was hyper-aware of the need to give my body the time—and care—to *truly* heal from the assault of surgery,

---

1 http://www.paintnite.com/

radiation, and emotional trauma. My post-cancer plan was a testament to joie de vivre: the joy of life.

I went to the home of my heart, Mexico, for six months. I stayed in a sweet little house on a hill called Casa Maraya with a spectacular view of the Bay of Banderas. I walked for hours and became stronger by climbing the steep hill 'home' everyday. I slept in if I needed to. I found an amazing modern-day "medicine woman" named Mari. Friends and family came to visit, and I cooked delicious organic meals for them infused with love. I made new friends. I wrote articles for local papers and joined a writer's group. I took Spanish classes with a lovely girl named Cecilia at an outdoor café. On weekends, I sold my books in the colorful farmer's markets. I whale-watched with delight. I hired a personal trainer twice a week for $7 a session. I played. And I did not need a windfall to do these things. I knew in my heart that I needed a period of time après cancer that was one of pure joy.

I urge you to allow yourself the time to do the same—to do the things that you know would be your ultimate medicine. It is the gift of a lifetime.

Far too often we live our lives counter to what we know is best for our health and happiness. Do you hear cancer's counsel?

Here is a statement to write on the mirror: *I give myself permission to take perfect care of myself.*

9

Work

"No one on their deathbed ever says they wish they had spent more time at the office."
—Paul Tsongas

There are people who choose to work through the experience of cancer. From my observations, it is frequently a decision based on the need to distract oneself from the pain and fear. However, your body just gave you a glaring notification. Placing undue stress and demands on your system as it persistently works overtime to heal is not in your best interests.

Cancer is a call from your soul if you choose to listen. Instead of distracting yourself by working, embrace your feelings. They may be overwhelming right now, but they will pass. I promise. Most cancer hospitals offer meditation classes. The techniques provided will greatly alleviate your angst.

If you absolutely need a distraction, volunteer to walk a dog, read to a child, or visit the elderly. Helping others when you are in need yourself can bring a sense of empowerment. You could also take a light online course or a class you have been itching to attend.

Most jobs offer decent health benefits for time off work, especially for cancer. The first time I was diagnosed I was paid 66% of my wage and I had support from my spouse.

The second time the story was very different. I was single and working contractually. I had no benefits and I was unable to get them privately because of the first diagnosis. The company I had worked with for many years decided to replace me due to the unknown amount of time off that I required. Within two weeks I had been given a diagnosis and a "pink slip." Had I said I could work through the treatments, I would have been able to stay. Knowing from firsthand experience what lay ahead, I had no such impulse.

It did cause me severe financial hardship and my savings were wiped out at mid-life. I was in no position to be out of work without benefits, but I did what was best for my healing and ultimately, my sanity and my life.

If you are considering working through cancer, be aware of your motives. Some people consider it a sign of superhumanness, but from the perspective of someone who has given a huge amount of contemplative time on what life is all about—*it ain't about the office.*

If you have a wonderful business or career that feeds your soul and brings you joy, fine. However, if you are under the heavy demands of management, reconsider. If there is any possible way to take the time off, do so. Treat your beloved body with the respect and love that it deserves as it fights to heal. It will in turn be in a position to bring you back to equilibrium.

There will always be a full inbox, something to finish, and an urgent matter. It can all wait.

10

Finances

"I finally know what distinguishes man from other beasts:
financial worries."
—Jules Renard

Cancer can take a massive financial toll. Fortunately in Canada we have a medical system that covers a good portion of conventional treatments. However, there can be extra costs for exorbitant prescriptions and if you are self-employed, there is the burden of dealing with regular obligations while taking time off. Also, most alternative treatments are not covered unless you have a specialized health plan.

Most Canadians assume that if they ever needed help, they would get it. Because of the heavy fundraising and awareness campaigns, we especially believe this to be true with breast cancer. The big 'Pink Ribbon' people—one being the Canadian Breast Cancer Foundation—allot absolutely nothing to breast cancer patients who need financial help. Just to give you an idea, revenues in the prairies alone for 2011 were over $12 million.

I applied to Canada Pension's Disability program. With my doctor's report, I was told that for all intents and purpose, I had cancer light, I would likely live, and I would be fine—not approved.

The local cancer social worker had only almost nothing to offer. If you have savings and/or have RRSPs (retirement savings) you are not eligible for funds. Years of diligence investing dollar-by-dollar will actually penalize anyone requiring assistance. Until you are in this position, you would not know that a lifetime Canadian citizen is not entitled to assistance.

There are some grants available through privately funded foundations, but it can take a lot of work to find them. If you are too tired to deal with it, have someone do the research on your behalf if you require financial assistance.

The current craze on raising money during an illness is crowdfunding.

If you need assistance, have someone set up a page for you on sites like GoFundMe[1].

Here is some basic advice for crowdfunding should you decide to go this route:

- Be sure to tell your story clearly and positively.
- Be imaginative and design the campaign with current graphic trends.
- Gain the support of friends and family immediately upon launching. It will be hard to get strangers onboard if your friends and family won't support your cause.
- Use social media to get the word out quickly and ask friends to share.
- Communicate with supporters. Be certain to send a thank you and an update.
- Have someone create a short, articulate video explaining what you are asking for and why.
- Get help creating a campaign inexpensively using Fiverr.com (search 'crowdfunding campaigns').

In the USA, The Patient Advocate Foundation and LIVESTRONG[2] have partnered to help cancer patients deal with medical debt.

---

1   https://www.gofundme.com/
2   http://www.livestrong.org/wecanhelp

11

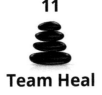

Team Heal

"I would rather walk with a friend in the dark, than alone in the light."
—Helen Keller

Now is the time to let people help. Cancer is a busy world—one that you need to tame. You may feel overwhelmed by appointments, tests, and well-wishers and you will have an easier time with assistance. I have always been a highly independent soul, but I learned that when I need help, I must let people be of service. Most people want to contribute, so remember that it also helps them to help you.

I worked at a demanding sales job when I was diagnosed in the summer of 1990 and I also had a side-business designing jewelry. I had booked and paid for *The Fringe Festival*, a lucrative ten-day gig for my jewelry biz. Friends stepped up and offered to take shifts at my booth so that I didn't have to cancel and lose the booth fee and the extra income. And I let them. They had fun selling my wares and it was no hardship for them.

The day I received the verdict on my second diagnosis is deeply etched in my mind (as is likely the same with you). I was obsessed as I awaited the call. Time dragged on interminably and so I finally called the doctor's office. As it turned out, my family doctor was away on vacation. I was driving down a highway returning home from an afternoon of sales calls when my phone rang. It was one of my doctor's colleagues calling with the report. I remember pulling over, my heart pounding out of my chest.

I had not told anyone in my family about the situation because I had not wanted to worry them needlessly. They had been through enough with me. For weeks, I held the secret and now the results were in. The doctor, not knowing me, had little sensitivity when she casually told me, "It's cancer."

Alone in my car on the side of a highway, I fell apart. When I say, "fell apart," I mean a code red, full-scale meltdown. After I regained a modicum of composure, I called two friends and asked them to come to my apartment after work. When you are with family and friends, threats become a little less menacing. Isolation at a time like this could be disastrous.

Single this time, I opted to go back to my home city for surgery so that I would be able to recuperate at my mum's and have her magnificent mother-hen care, and be surrounded by old friends who had been through this with me before.

I would like to offer a small forewarning. Friends may not respond to your diagnosis as you would expect. Some people cannot give you the type of support you need. An important thing to understand is that people will not always react to your illness according to your beliefs and needs, they will respond according to *theirs*. Some are afraid; others do not have a clue what to say; while some just cannot handle the cancer scene. Please try not to take it personally.

I have a friend who doesn't believe in illness and so she couldn't or wouldn't be with me in the way I requested.

When I was in the hospital on my first go 'round, one of my closest friends came to see me and demanded that I take off my bandage to show her my fresh lumpectomy scar. Thankfully an astute nurse came into the room and put a stop to her badgering. Then she asked if she could get the key to my house so that she could borrow a dress for an upcoming wedding. It wasn't what I had expected from a close friend, but her belief was that this was a matter-of-fact situation.

On the other hand, I received an onslaught of support that I could not have imagined.

Three dear friends showed up late one evening with a plaid tablecloth and a picnic basket full of fabulous food and we feasted on my hospital bed. I have never forgotten that special night.

A client-turned-friend brought calamari and tzatziki from my favorite Greek restaurant.

Another friend I had not seen in years showed up with the biggest balloon bouquet I had ever seen.

A colleague I had worked with years earlier sent me a spray of stupendous long-stemmed roses.

People called to ask if I would permit their church groups to pray for me.

I was offered meals, house cleaning, and all types of assistance. Some I really did not need, but if it made the experience easier, I gratefully accepted. Allow people to keep your healing space clean, orderly, and pretty if they offer. It clears the mind.

As I mentioned before, if you are too overwhelmed, assign your research to others. You can forward information from this book or any other sources that you wish to learn about. Ask them to create a concise document of information for you.

Ask people to accompany you to appointments. It can be scary to go for scans and tests and if you have someone to lighten your mood it makes the time pass more quickly and easily.

For the more private, it can be tempting to hide yourself away from others because of the pain you are feeling and the extreme vulnerability you are experiencing. But know that people are not judging you. They are not feeling as sorry for you as you think. They are awed by your courage and they are inspired by your journey.

Men, if you are inclined to suffer in silence and bottle your emotions, please let this be the time you open up with your friends and family. Your significant other cannot carry the whole burden of this challenge. Talk to your closest friends about how you feel. Men need support from their brothers and have the right to ask for assistance.

Let people help. Don't isolate. You do not have to take this journey as a stoic pillar. Allow others to show their love. It is a healing force and truly feels good.

12

Connection. Groups. Therapy.

"Sometimes, reaching out and taking someone's hand is the beginning of a journey. At other times, it is allowing another to take yours."
—Vera Nazarian

One of the fundamental necessities of a human being is a sense of connection. It is what gives life significance. Statistics reveal that people have a higher cure rate going through cancer when they have support. The type of support you need to thrive is a personal preference.

Writer and researcher Dan Buettner studied human longevity and wrote about it in the book called *The Blue Zones*. The "Blue Zones" are regions in the world where people live the longest and remain robust and active late in life. In his findings, one of the key factors for a long, productive, and healthy life was distinctly connected to a strong sense of community. People who look out for each other and bond on a daily basis are healthier and live longer.

What I have learned in my travels is the art of sensual and slow living with a strong social connection. I have joined Mexicans as they cluster around taco stands and socialize. I enjoyed a two-hour high tea in Buenos Aires with new friends. I slowly savored four-course meals mid-day in Oaxaca with the locals. In Cuba, I was constantly pulled onto the dance floor in small bars in Old Havana with an alliance of music lovers. My friend and I participated in the *Italiano* tradition of bonding at tiny corner wine bars for a glass of vino after their workday ended in Florence. When I'm in Vallarta, I frequently bump into friends or even strangers on the street and make spontaneous coffee dates that last for hours. Here in Canada, people are typically scheduled well in advance and sadly spontaneity has become almost extinct.

Wherever I go, I try to build some type of community. It was a blow when I lost the coffee shop camaraderie I had built over a 15-year span in my old neighborhood because the café was taken over by a fast food chain. I had relationships with all of the sweet baristas that worked there over the years and they and many of the patrons were my writing fans. I still miss the kinship I had with my neighbors in the antiquated walk-up apartment I lived in for 16 years long after I was flooded out and had to move. We could count on each other for almost anything and we took care of each other. Find your tribe, wherever it may be right now.

Support groups are available for almost anything. I attended a few different cancer group sessions, but did not find they were suitable for me. People tended to focus on a victim mentality and on their conditions, protocols, and problems. I needed a positive and uplifting environment and gave up on support groups. That is not to say you won't find a group with a good attitude that will work well for you, but if you don't feel elevated, you may wish to seek something different. Commiserating in misery is not the best way to deal with cancer. What I did find in these groups was the confirmation that support, love, and care from friends and family is of utmost importance. The people who did not have any suffered the most.

A church or spiritual center can be a perfect place to find solace and support. If you do not have one and want to attend, ask friends where they go and why. Ritual and prayer both with others and in solitude is helpful through cancer to help quell fear.

There are other ways to find a sense of connection and community. Group art therapy, creative journaling classes, ceramics, and music classes are frequently offered at cancer foundations and support centers, as well as gentle yoga, meditation, and movement classes. Friendships can be formed in these caring groups. You may find what you are looking for on MeetUp.com as well.

There is healing power in psychological therapy during and after cancer. The first time, I was assigned a psychologist at the cancer institute and he did not seem to understand what I was going through as a young newlywed with a cancer diagnosis, so I asked for a reassignment. I was matched with a feisty little Irish psychologist who fit my personality perfectly. She worked well with my then-husband too.

The second time I had cancer I met with a psychologist for a few sessions. I soon realized that the diagnosis had thrown me into a spiritual crisis and a serious fury with my "Maker." I was connected with a wonderful and warm spiritual therapist named Bert. She was a source of solace and I saw her long past the cancer treatments. When you feel like no one understands your journey, a therapist can offer a compassionate presence. He or she can lend an ear to listen to your innermost fears, your anger, and your doubts. You can discuss your feelings and plans without bias and receive calm guidance.

You will also find trained volunteers who are usually survivors and they will meet up for one-on-one support through your experience. When I was 29 it seemed as if everyone going through cancer was either a small child or a senior. If you can, find those your age who are going through cancer so that you can relate to each other.

Nobody should face cancer alone. Be sure to seek connection during your journey.

No Man's an Island
09/13/2014

"We cannot live only for ourselves. A thousand fibers connect us with our fellow men; and among those fibers, as sympathetic threads, our actions run as causes, and they come back to us as effects."
—Herman Melville

I know I have an advantage when it comes to connecting with strangers because I am single (and have been since the Neolithic Age). I have no distractions or people demanding things of me. I also wander about life solo a good portion of the time and connecting assuages my occasional feelings of aloneness.

Oprah maintains that in all of the interviews she has done and stories she has shared, the one common denominator in all people, be they Beyoncé Knowles or a murderer on death row, is that we all want to be seen. Do we matter? Do we count? Are we heard? With that innate need seeded in all of us, alienation and being ignored or overlooked can be the death of our spirit.

Aside of my wanderlust, one of the driving forces for my goal of living in cultures that have underlying foundations of rich human connection is to leave behind a city that fosters anonymity. But no matter where I am, the other advantage I hold is that I am open to connection. I seek it. And it enriches my life in ways that exceed worldly goods.

I went for a cherished bi-summer pedicure last month and brought in my laptop to do some writing since my Vietnamese guy-pedicurist is a silent type. His precocious 6 year-old daughter was in the salon that day. She was rather taken with me because I apparently have hair similar to Elsa the Snow Queen in the movie *Frozen*. I was soon to learn she is obsessed with *Frozen*.

She wanted to know what I was writing and so I showed her one of my websites and some of my gift books. She began picking books off the shelf.

"Did you write this book?"

"No."

"This one?"

"Ah ... no."

"How about this one?"

"Nope."

She sat next to me and narrated the entire tale of *Frozen*.

"Okay. Now write it," she instructed.

"I think I best see the movie before I write the book to get it all straight," I said.

"Let's look at *Frozen* on YouTube!" she said.

"Okay, I can do that."

I pulled up the theme song and asked her if she wanted to sing it.

"Yes! Yes!" she said, clapping her hands.

There we sat in the salon, belting out frozen fractals and *Let it Go, Let it Go*. She knew every word.

There is something about engaging with a child that makes you joyfully lose your inhibitions and enter their twinkling world. I did not get to write a word, but I left with a refreshed heart.

Another day I was in the chic boutique, Value Village (if you say 'village' with a French accent it sounds impressive), looking at skirts. An Asian woman with a deep accent came up to me with two knapsacks. She wanted to know which one I thought was best for an upcoming ocean cruise with her husband. I could see she was extremely excited about this maiden voyage. I told her which one I thought was best and why.

Again, she came up and asked another question about the bags. I reiterated why my first choice was the better and gave her some more features and benefits.

"For $3.99, you can't go wrong."

She then began to look at clothing with me. I found this amusing since she was considerably smaller than I. She held up a black flowing skirt.

"This would be nice for cruise, yes?"

I laughed. "Yes it would, but I think you'd find it on the floor. It's far too big for you. You need to look over there in the petite section," I pointed.

"Yes, I know. Thing is, I just want to be near you," she said in her heavily accented English. "You have good taste. You nice!"

When we lend an ear and share in the excitement of another, we reap the reward of a momentary flash of friendship.

One sunny day I went to the park after work to lollygag and bond with Mother Nature. After I had gotten myself set up, I noticed that my red blanket and fuchsia top artistically matched the lush circle of flowers next to me.

As I lay reading Fast Forward Magazine, I heard some young Aboriginal people walking up behind me.

"Hey …. there's Anna, that women who died … Anna Smith something."

"No it's not," said the girl. "It's Dolly Parton."

I giggled behind my paper. Thank you, Victoria's Secret.

One of the young men stopped.

"I'm going to stay here for a minute. You guys go ahead."

He turned to me.

"Do you mind if I sit down and talk to you?"

"No."

"So … you died. Then you came back. Why'd you come back?"

I went with it.

"Well, sometimes you gotta come back and check things out."

"Mmm hmm. So," he said in all seriousness, "What's it like?"

"Awesome! Fabulous!"

"Good. I think I'm ready to go."

"Why?"

"Well, I drink a lot, you know. The doctor told me my liver's really bad and I'm going to die."

"Have you thought about maybe quitting and sticking around Earth?"

"Awww, I don't know. Maybe … You look so young laying there."

I *love* gravity, I thought to myself.

"Your eyes are freaking me out. I've never seen eyes like that. I almost can't look at you," he said as he covered his eyes with a hand.

"Don't be freaked out. They're only eyes."

I realized that for one thing, he'd likely only ever looked into brown eyes. For another, I'd guessed no white woman with green eyes had ever looked deeply into his. (However, in Native culture it is the norm to avoid prolonged eye contact out of respect, so this may have been a factor.)

We chattered a little more.

Then his friend came up and said it was time to go. He got up, shook my hand, and thanked me for the conversation.

As they got near their car, I heard him say to his buddy, "That was Anna Nicole Smith!"

"No it isn't. It's Marilyn Monroe."

How beautiful we may look to people of other origins. Possibly I gave him the gift of listening, but he gave me the sweet gift of seeing myself as something I don't catch much in the mirror anymore.

On the long weekend I went for a walk along the river. My friend Francis had introduced me to a couple who live along the path. They were outside, so I stopped to say hello. They kindly invited me to join them for a drink. He is a transplant surgeon and she is a pathologist, both from another country. Their son was cooking and I was invited to join them for a light al fresco dinner.

They are intelligent conversationalists and good listeners. They asked many questions with sincerity. With this unplanned encounter, they gave me the gift of being seen and heard on a very solo weekend.

If we are open to it, sometimes we can be the bridge of an amazing connection for others. I'm not usually the person who assists others in a big way, but because of my years in sales, I'm prone to promoting others.

In 2007 I took two wondrous one-month trips to Oaxaca, Mexico filled with interesting people and experiences. Within my first two hours in Oaxaca, I met a young waiter named Abimael. He asked if I would like to trade English lessons for Spanish lessons and I thought it was a brilliant idea. We would sit in *Oaxaqueño* coffee shops and study one hour of English then one hour of Spanish.

He accompanied me on fascinating day trips to outlying Indigenous villages and went with me to see a strange medicine woman for a skin condition that I wanted to heal.

Abi was getting an English degree to teach and desperately wanted to come to Canada to further learn in an English-speaking country. I live in a one-bedroom apartment so could not offer accommodations, but I set out to help him find a place to stay. I mentioned it in conversation with my sister. Soon she was plotting how she could help make it happen. She decided to invite him into her own home for the six-month visit.

I certainly wasn't the Earth angel, but I did connect Abi with one.

My sister not only hosted him for free (no charge for *anything*), she took him with her family on road trips, introduced him to friends, found an English tutor, and helped him get a job earning more money than he had ever seen in his life. She was happy with the much-needed positive male influence he gave to her two young sons with his even mood, steady smile, and easy laughter.

We catch a hit of that delectable bonding hormone, oxytocin, when we share positive emotion. We get it at weddings, when someone sings the national anthem, during a standing ovation, and when we watch glorious creatures such as dolphins playing or whales breaching. We get it when we find ourselves in fascinating (usually unexpected) conversations or sharing any magnificent moment.

We can all give someone the honor of being seen and heard. It might be a stranger in a café, a colleague, or someone in our own home whom we have taken for granted or think we know fully. Even if our lives are busy, we can always take the time to flash a smile, give a compliment, or chat in a line. We can make our own day by making another's.

People are good at putting up façades. We have no idea what someone is struggling with inside (Robin Williams showed us that), so if you hear a little voice telling you to connect, follow through. It just may be someone's guardian angel asking.

Our hearts swell a little when we connect with others—it's because it's a crazy little thing called love.

An amazing display of human connection! (Tissues required)
Homeless Shelter Surprise: http://youtu.be/r-8ee7qyfF0

No Man's an Island:
http://wp.me/p2ACw4-qf
lifebyheart.wandasthilaire.com

13

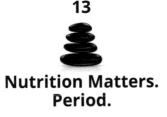

Nutrition Matters.
Period.

"The planet Earth is one of the greatest pharmacies ever invented.
And we're ignoring most of it."
—Dr. Patrick Quillin

When I asked the oncologists about nutrition, I was told to eat whatever I wanted. But, disease begins with cellular imbalances, and poor eating habits can be the tipping point. I cannot fathom why most doctors—society's modern-day healers—are *still* not given proper information and education on nutrition and the effects of food on the body (although, as previously stated, I am aware that pharmaceutical funding and patriarchal control has a lot to do with this issue). The evidence of this can be found in hospitals all over North America; the food served in their cafeterias and to their patients is preposterously lacking in proper nutrition and imagination.

In spite of endlessly compelling research and data, education on nutrition in the medical model, in essence, does not exist. We now have an enormous amount of clinical research and information at our fingertips about food and the myriad ways it impacts our health. Food can help heal cancer.

However, pharmaceutical and surgical intervention can be quicker when someone is in a health crisis. Also, physicians know from experience it is sometimes harder to get a patient to change their food habits than to get them to take a pill or treatment. In a discussion with my doctor, she said more often than not, her patients' eyes glaze over when she touches on the subject of diet or exercise. Also, if a doctor is not personally following healthy eating habits themselves, they are not apt to preach it.

Eating processed, deep-fried, and fast food filled with an excess of trans fats, preservatives, MSG, sugar, and artificial flavors and colors (basically fake food with little to no nutritive value) is *not* going help you heal. This type of diet negatively impacts genetic expression. Healthy, whole foods can help your immune system fight any free roaming cancer cells, and boost your strength, while positively impacting genetic expression.

I am by no means a health-food fanatic. When the MD in Mexico put me on a strict diet, I almost cried. And, under such restriction, as I frequented the restaurants and cafés I love, I did cry. I have never been a dieter and I am an avid foodie. I love gourmet, wholesome, tasty food. I also love carbs and sauces. But, after a month of stringent cleansing, a high-nutrient diet, and natural treatments, I went home energetic and strong. I felt great and looked good. One of my friends was the operating room's head nurse when I had my lumpectomy; she told me that the anesthesiologist said I was strong and needed a smaller amount of anesthetic than normal. The surgery went quickly and without complication.

Food matters. You can kid yourself that you do not need to eat your greens, but that won't serve you. Bestselling author and wellness advocate Kris Carr has been living with stage IV cancer for over a decade— her "thrival" heavily influenced by a high nutrition diet, and health & cancer coach Chris Wark cured himself of stage III colon cancer (minus chemo) in 2003 through a radical diet change and natural non-toxic remedies. In 1991, 28-year old Glenn Sabin was diagnosed with incurable chronic lymphocytic leukemia. Through diet, complementary medicine, and lifestyle changes that were monitored by MDs, he *cured* his fatal cancer (minus chemo) and is a studied and documented case in medical literature.

Dr. David Servan-Schreiber, a physician and neuroscience researcher, discovered he had a tumor when a volunteer for a brain scan failed to show up for some research he was working on and he ended up under the scanner himself. It revealed a brain tumor that was cancerous.

He was successfully treated by conventional means and was told to go back to life as usual. He continued to eat and behave the same way as before. The cancer returned a few years later. With that second wake-up call, he began to research cancer prevention.

An expert in research and statistical data, he looked deeply into the healing power of food. In his book, *Anticancer: A New Way of Life*, he outlined a list of cancer-fighting and healing foods. The most basic vegetables and fruits found at your local grocery store
can have a significant impact on your health. The information in his

book provides a clear understanding of good nutrition and an extensive list of superfoods.

If you are not inclined to read the book, what follows are some simple, common sense guidelines. Do not panic (as I did). While you are going through treatment and beyond, you give yourself the best chance of success by supporting your body with life-affirming food. You need not fall into depression over the loss of your favorite foods. Your palate will change and cravings will dissipate. If your body is working overtime to clean up toxicity from a poor diet it has a harder time fighting cancer. Think of it like nutrition rocket fuel to kick cancer's ass.

It can be difficult to incorporate changes in your diet when everyone around you is munching on junk. If you live with others, ask them to join you. What I share below is also excellent advice for prevention of illness. Have your family support your efforts on the road to wellness through new eating habits and delicious, wholesome meals that will undoubtedly improve everyone's energy levels and long-term health.

- Almost everything in the produce section is plant-based and heals. Fill your cart here. Choose organic if you can afford it.
- Boxed foods with a long list of bizarre sounding ingredients are a poor choice for healing.
- Avoid all artificial sweeteners and MSG. Better choices are real maple syrup, honey, agave, or stevia.
- Himalayan sea salt has beneficial minerals and tastes great.
- Get good fats: coconut oil and coconut milk, avocado, fatty fish, chia seeds, olives, extra virgin olive oil, nuts, and natural nut butters.
- Avoid overloading your body with sugar and heavy white carbohydrates. Research shows that cancer loves processed white sugar so do not fill up on candy bars and sweet desserts to keep your weight from plummeting.
- Satiate chocolate cravings with raw organic cacao by adding it to smoothies, yogurt, or banana pancakes. Available in powder, butter, beans, and nibs, raw cacao is a superfood that is high in magnesium, chromium, antioxidants and various essential minerals. It is also an excellent mood and energy booster.
- Anything processed with imitation flavoring, chemical taste enhancers, and added coloring is not a healthy choice.
- Anything deep-fried is a very poor choice.

- Avoid trans fats and edible oil products such as margarine, fake cheese, coffee whiteners, commercial baked goods, and snack food. This is not real food.
- Any soda pop—*especially* diet pop—is a harmful choice for hydration.
- Clean, organic protein is important in healing tissue destroyed by radiation and chemotherapy.
- Limit caffeine and stop ingesting chemically laden energy drinks. Have herbal teas when possible.
- Avoid GMOs (genetically modified/engineered food).
- Fresh juice is highly nutritional and vitamin packed (best investment in your wellness plan: a good juicer).
- Green smoothies give you heaps of vitamins, fiber, and green content in one glass of goodness. There are countless recipes on Pinterest. I have included some of mine below.
- Drink lots and lots of clean water to detoxify and hydrate the cells.
- Adding sprouts gives you a huge nutritional boost: broccoli sprouts, alfalfa sprouts, radish sprouts, etc.
- If you can, add naturally fermented foods. They are an excellent source of probiotics and nutrients. Examples are homemade sauerkraut, dill carrots, kefir, fermented pickles, kimchi, kombucha, miso, tempeh, and fermented wheat germ extract.
- The four top cancer-fighting spices are turmeric, cayenne, garlic, and oregano.
- Superfoods with super high ORAC rating (measure of antioxidants): Sumac, Ceylon cinnamon, raw cacao, Indian gooseberries, pecans, turmeric, baobab fruit, red and black sorghum, chia seeds, and purple corn.
- Avoid microwave cooking. It destroys nutrients, especially in vegetables.

I recently stopped at a medi-center for a sinus/chest infection. When I'm not feeling well I tend to crave comfort food like macaroni and cheese and spaghetti or nutrition-empty food like canned tomato soup with crackers. It was the first time an MD told me to eat lots of fruits and vegetables to boost my immune system for an infection. She reminded me to make better choices. I believe I healed faster because I juiced and ate platefuls of greens and fruits.

A colleague/friend of mine has juiced every morning for the past 20 years. Even when she's on the road for business, she takes her juicer along and makes a concoction of carrot/beet/celery/kale/cucumber juice before going for a walk. She has never been in the hospital, never had a serious illness, and rarely gets sick from flu and cold bugs. She's a walking testament to the nutritive power of juicing.

If you do any research on nutrition and diet you will learn that a portion of the goal is to create an alkaline environment in the body. Cancer appears to thrive in an acidic body. Fruits and vegetables alkalize the body and help reduce inflammation.

Both times while undergoing radiation, I madly craved protein and I ate even more than normal. I did not become temporarily anorexic (as can happen) and did not lose weight during treatments. As I previously mentioned, my skin did not burn and I did not develop lymphedema.

I was also told it was okay to drink alcohol. A glass of wine or a beer now and then is not going to crash your system, but drinking on a regular basis through treatments may suppress immunity and tax your liver.

Again (because so many people avoid water), be sure to keep yourself well hydrated with clean water. Add fresh lemons or limes for a tasty health boost. Aim for 6-8 glasses per day.

We typically think of blessing our food as a religious act. Possibly you already do this. On the other hand, it may be a radical concept for you, but this is not just a religious idea; if you are aware that everything is energy, then saying thank you or blessing a meal is an act of generating positive energy.

I adored the Mexican movie, *Like Water For Chocolate*, which illustrates this concept powerfully. It is a magical realism tale of how our emotions affect the food we prepare. When I cook with love and appreciation, I have proven that my meals taste far better than when I am mind-numbed, in a hurry, or especially if I am angry.

There is a huge benefit to integrating sensual joys in your life and eating should be pleasurable. If you have been at war with food, stressing yourself out by counting calories, or carbs, or fats, or obsessing—stop, forevermore. Make peace with eating. If you eat only to survive, investigate the joy of eating good food.

With the surge of interest in health and nutrition, the variety of delicious recipes that can be found for nutrient-rich cancer-healing meals is staggeringly awesome. Think of counting colors on your plate as a way to monitor your intake of goodness (reds, varying greens, yellows, oranges, deep purples, etc.). You will be surprised at how quickly your craving for junk dissipates. Flood your body with living food.

A few years ago, I met a food writer from Hawaii at a writer's conference in San Miguel de Allende. Fast forward and we recently had dinner when she pit-stopped in Canada. I was stunned when she pulled out the draft of her new book, *Kicking Cancer*. Ironically, she is publishing her book at the same time as I am publishing mine, and we have both had breast cancer. She told me that when she had the lumpectomy twenty years ago, the doctors could not believe the cancer had not metastasized due to the size of the tumor, so they removed a whopping twenty-nine of her lymph nodes. This caused a lot of swelling, drainage of lymphatic fluid, and overall malaise.

Since she was not recovering well enough for radiation, a friend sent her to a naturopathic doctor, who in turn revamped her supplement regime and put her on a high nutrition diet. Within *48 hours* she noticed a marked difference. The experience set her on a path to study preventative nutrition and inspired her to create delicious, healthy recipes. She, too, believes food should not be eaten if it doesn't taste great. Twenty years later she is alive and not only well, but a vivacious woman who looks far younger than she is. She is fully living her passion in panoramic color, writing and traveling. Her new book is a cornucopia of delectable, life-giving recipes, and nutritive information.

If you are not prone to making a drastic shift in your diet, make healthy choices that will help you on your healing journey and keep you strong. Many researchers in this field believe food is medicine and multitudes of people have healed their cancer by diet alone. It is up to you how far you want to take it. Remember, natural food downregulates faulty genes and you cannot overdose on good nutrition.

And please do not self-medicate with recreational drugs while going through any type of surgery or treatments. Medical marijuana and hemp oil, as prescribed by a professional, which can help with pain and is curative falls outside the category of self-medication. Also, if you smoke, you know what to do, A.S.A.P. If need be, seek hypnotherapy to assist you in quitting.

Meals are an area where friends and family can be tremendously helpful, especially if you are used to dining out a lot. If someone asks you what they can do for you, have them shop and juice, prepare fruits for smoothies, or make you healthy meals (not a bunch of carb and fat-laden casseroles please!).

If you are not feeling well, smoothies are a fantastic way to bump up the nutrition without choking down platefuls of food. I am including three of my favorite creations, plus a detoxifying green drink. I cube fruit and freeze it for a quick and easy smoothie. It is best to freeze fruit on a cookie sheet first and then place it in freezer bags or glass jars so that it doesn't clump together.

I like the first one in the morning because it is filling and creamy like a milkshake.

The avocado contains the perfect oil for your body and gives the smoothie its rich consistency. If you need to increase your caloric intake due to weight loss, replace almond milk with coconut milk or coconut cream. If you have access to fresh young coconuts, add it to your smoothies. Get extra calories through natural drinks, *not* processed canned drinks.

Wanda's Morning Smoothie

- Unsweetened almond milk (best brand for taste: Almond Breeze)
- ½ of a small or ¼ of a large avocado
- One small or ½ of a large frozen banana
- Spinach (handful of raw)
- English cucumber (2" slice cubed)
- Optional protein boost: Organic ground raw hemp (unflavored)
- A few good shakes of cinnamon

Creamy Bliss Smoothie

This one is very simple, filling, and tastes fantastic.

- One small or ½ of a large frozen banana
- Unsweetened almond milk (vanilla, plain, or almond-coconut blend)
- Papaya (handful of cubes frozen or fresh)
- ½ of an avocado

Afternoon Health Burst Smoothie

- Filtered water
- Lemon (juice of a whole lemon)
- Spinach (large handful)
- Apple (½ or whole for larger smoothie)
- Frozen banana (½ or whole for larger smoothie)
- ¼ English cucumber
- Celery (1–2 sticks)
- Variation choice: Handful of pineapple, kiwi, or pear cubes

Option for all smoothies: add a heaping tablespoon of ground flaxseed for fiber.

Excellent Detox Green Drink

(Drink in 5-day intervals off and on)
   This doesn't sound good, but it is. I served it at a family dinner and they fought over the last drops!

- Filtered water
- Ice
- Handful of cilantro (cilantro detoxes heavy metals)
- Handful of fresh mint leaves
- ¼ English cucumber
- Lemon (juice of a whole lemon)
- Couple of dashes of real maple syrup

Gentle Liver Detox

- Juice a full head of organic celery stalks until finished (make again) and drink once every second day for 2 weeks.

Easy Peasy Nutrition-Packed Pancakes

I created these pancakes one day and have been hooked ever since. They are quick and easy and are also wheat-free.

- One ripe banana, mashed (a potato masher works well)
- Two eggs
- Walnuts (substitute your favorite nuts or seeds)
- Cinnamon
- 2 heaping tablespoons of ground oats. Substitute almond flour, buckwheat flour, oat flour, or spelt flour to thicken.
- If you prefer pancakes with more density, add a heaping tablespoon of chia seeds and let sit for 10 minutes. They swell and are a healthy energy booster.
- If you're a chocolate lover, add a heaping teaspoon of raw cacao.

Stir well. Make mini pancakes in 1 full tablespoon of melted organic cold-pressed virgin coconut oil. These are great plain or with fresh mango slices or raspberries and plain Bio-Best yogurt (90% lactose free) with a drizzle of real maple syrup.

Here are some guidelines for understanding scanning stickers on conventionally grown (using pesticides, herbicides and fertilizers), organically grown and GMO (genetically modified) produce:

- Organically grown has five numbers that begin with a 9.
- Conventionally grown produce has 4 numbers only. The number 3 or 4 indicates conventionally grown.
- GMO produce has five numbers that begin with 8. Avoid all GMOs.

If you want to learn more about nutrition in an entertaining way, watch Drew Canole, on YouTube at *FitLifeTV*[1]. He's inspiring!

---

1   https://www.youtube.com/user/fitlifetv

14

The Antidote to Fear is Trust

I fear this jungle
For I know not whether with the turn of a leaf
I will find a deadly poisonous snake
Or an exquisitely beautiful butterfly
—Wanda St. Hilaire
Of Love, Life and Journeys

Fear is a major factor in the cancer journey, and I've had many moments of abject terror. In a hindsight review of my journal, *The Catalyst Chronicles*, I saw the incredible number of nightmares I had during Cancer II; ones containing tsunamis, tornadoes, fires, and plane crashes. Thankfully, I survived them all.

Avoidance or denial will not diminish fear at its roots. With cancer, we need to face what is. We fear suffering and we fear death.

There is a lot of talk about "hope" when the topic of cancer comes up. Hope is important, but sometimes feels more like a fingers-crossed approach.

Trust is something completely different. Trust allows you to open to an inner stillness, and is a requirement if you are to retain any semblance of calm. If it feels as if there is no predictability right now, suspend disbelief and embrace trust. Whatever your beliefs, drawing strength from and having confidence in the benevolence of a higher mind, the Universe, or God will help you traverse the ups and downs of the cancer experience. When you trust, there is a lightness of being.

My wise woman acupuncturist once told me in a session that when I was afraid, the antidote to fear was trust. Trust means having faith that what is happening is for a reason and that life knows what it's doing.

I hope you have begun to chart a wellness plan and are implementing it. You are taking care of yourself in the best way you know how. Now is the time to make peace with cancer. Now it is the time to trust.

Live every day in the emotion of victory.

The Eensy Weensy Spider
09/07/2012

"Promise me you'll always remember: you're braver than you believe, and stronger than you seem, and smarter than you think."
—Christopher Robin to Pooh Bear

On a recent sunny Saturday, a daddy longlegs took a detour into my picnic basket at the park and back at my apartment, began making its way across my hardwood floor. I watched it dart about, deciding which direction to take. I have a no kill policy; live and let live, but fear overtook compassion. I grabbed a shoe and flattened the poor thing.

I stood there for a long moment feeling bad (and grossed out) and saw the metaphor for the world's biggest problems in my arachnophobia. Rather than live harmoniously with what we fear, we want to kill or eradicate what we fear. On a grand scale, we have all seen what fear has done to the world.

As my acupuncturist "Obi" says, the antidote to fear is trust. As the spider wandered about, I had visions of it making its way across a shoulder while I read on the couch or maybe crawling across my face while I slept. If I could have trusted that this innocent creature would make its way out of my home or have found a suitable place to hang out, I would have let it be.

Three things occurred following the spider murder that brought the issue of trust loudly into my field of vision.

Firstly, I attended an evening at a friend's constellation workshop. This is a bizarro world healing modality with sometimes amazing results. I have been to a number of these and had agreed to attend in support of another friend who was going for the first time.

Much to my surprise, I was asked to participate in the lead role. As the session went on, it became apparent that the topic of the healing was pertinent in my own life; it was centered on the melding of one woman's heart and body with her life's purpose. The healing came in her agreement to shed the things that were keeping her from living her purpose.

I am unsure of what specific context in the constellation triggered it, but I later pondered why—for a girl who *loves* love—my love life in the past few years has become non-existent and a sentence flashed clearly in my mind about my level of trust in the realm of romantic relationships.

The second thing was a book. Two years ago, a friend lent me *The Shack*. I am an avid reader, but I have sidestepped that book on my shelf upon each perusal, refusing to read something that begins with the murder of a child. This time while scanning my collection of books, I singled it out and began to read.

In it, I discovered some very acceptable answers that go back to the "sweet" surrender I discussed in a previous post[1]. Why, I have asked myself, should I wholly surrender and "blindly" trust in light of the path my life has taken?

In a scene with the lead character, a highly comforting explanation about life is given, contrary to my early indoctrination, that there is not a malevolent and mean-spirited being exacting punishment arbitrarily (with things like cancer) or smiting us for entertainment. The web of the Universe holds a neutral field of love.

Another is that if we relinquish our stubborn stance of independence and consider walking in hopeful expectation with ourselves and with our higher power (whatever or whomever that may be) with openness and at least a pinch of trust, then the falls we take and the hardships we endure just might not be as grueling as when we plod alone.

One line that radically resonated for me was, "It's extremely hard to rescue someone unless he is willing to trust you."

The freedom comes in the friendship with the divine.

The third thing that happened was a profound class at school about exploring the thoughts and actions behind success. We first watched a Ted Talk with an amazing woman named Caroline Casey called 'Looking Past Limits[2]' and look past limits this woman has done. The amount of trust Caroline Casey has in herself and in life, in spite of a considerable limitation, will boggle your mind.

The filter that we see the world through starts forming by what we hear, see, feel and experience as young children. As we navigate through life, each significant experience and event further shapes our

---

1   Sweet Surrender – http://wp.me/p2ACw4-4f
2   http://blog.ted.com/2011/04/08/looking-past-limits-caroline-casey-on-ted-com/

beliefs. If something negative (or something we believe to be negative) or traumatic occurs, we are likely unaware of how our view of the world insidiously alters according to the impact to our hearts, lives, and our emotional states.

We do not spend time thinking about our levels of trust. Until we intimately discussed our business goals in relation to our underlying beliefs in class, I had never stopped to consider whether I had a high degree of trust or not, never mind how that might be impinging on the results in my life.

In *The Spontaneous Healing of Belief*[1], Gregg Braden says that our deepest, biggest core belief which shapes our ultimate experience of life boils down to one big Kahuna question: do we believe in a beneficent, kind Universe looking out for our best interests or do we believe that the world is out to crap on us at every turn? (That might be a paraphrase.)

After the Ted Talk, Selena, our instructor/coach, asked the difficult questions with a few light bulb moments igniting in the room. In my own microcosm, I became aware of being a "ye of little faith" kind of girl as of late. I realized four monumental distrusts I am harboring.

I do not completely trust my body because of its maladies in spite of my best efforts at health.

I do not trust romance because of all the rascals and rogues I have lusted and loved over the course of my life.

I do not fully trust myself because of some messy mistakes I have made.

But most of all, I do not really trust divinity because of the dark and pain-filled falls I have taken, sometimes leaping into free fall with faith and landing in agonizing face-plants.

Basically Mr. Braden, I would have to say that I have been trying to dodge the flying crap.

If one does not trust life, how can life give us the beauty we seek?

And so, as one would fundamentally need living life by heart, I planted the idea of trusting in life once again. Just like Jack's magic beanstalk, that teeny tiny seedling has begun to grow rather rapidly. (What was that about the mustard seed?)

Small leaves are starting to sprout. Cool happenstances are cropping up. The wind is rustling and swirling with a slight scent of possibility.

---

1 http://www.greggbraden.com/about-gregg-braden

But the biggest and best in this new experiment of trust—for a girl who loves love—is that I fulfilled one of my 'Manifesto' wishes within a week. At Expo Latino, my favorite event of the year, I said a whole-hearted *yes* to dancing into the wee hours (*la madrugada*) of the night and found myself in a series of bodacious joy spots (no, I didn't say G spots!) that I have not been in for many years.

That slice of the pie chart in another post[1], the Joy-Play-Adventure piece, with a dash of trust, expanded exponentially in the wink of an eye.

P.S. Please don't miss Caroline Casey's inspiring TedTalk 'Looking Past Limits'

https://youtu.be/YyBk55G7Keo

The Eensy Weensy Spider
http://wp.me/p2ACw4-8n
lifebyheart.wandasthilaire.com

1   Where's the Mother Ship? – http://wp.me/p2ACw4-60

15

Stress

Rushing and running
Confused little beings
Caught in a maze
Schedules, deadlines, obligations
Furrowed brows and migraines
Tempers stretched; igniting
Futile obscenities screamed in traffic
How bewildered God must be
as he watches us dash past love, truth, and beauty
—Wanda St. Hilaire
Of Love, Life and Journeys

I have done it. My friends do it. My sister does it. We excuse insane stress levels for the sake of something—our jobs, our kids, our dis-functional relationships. We will do something about it soon. We will take some time off. We will start disciplining the kids next week. But we cannot afford the "luxury" of living in a constant state of stress or unhappiness. The body's immune defense mechanisms dial down when we are under duress and sprint through life.

The amygdala signals the stress response, which fills the body with an excess of toxic hormones. The body shuts down the immune system to conserve energy in defense against the danger it perceives; the threat generated by anxiety. The blood vessels in the stomach squeeze tight, impeding digestion and creating a sensation of nervous butterflies and indigestion (and sometimes constipation or diarrhea). The production of healthy cells is significantly compromised. When we relax, the repair system and immunity mechanisms for disease and infection switch back on. The stomach once again functions normally.

Scientists confirm that stress is the leading cause of disease. Dr. Bruce Lipton (father of epigenetics) cites that 90% of illness is caused by stress.

It does not take a scientist to see the negative effects of tension on our bodies and our mental wellness. Many of us are in a perpetual state of fight-or-flight without even knowing it.

When we are in stress mode, our bodies secrete an excess of cortisol, a hormone that can be worse for our health than smoking. Cortisol causes a dangerous increase in weight around the stomach. Drastic peaks and dips during the day shrink the hippocampus, our emotional regulation system. We make poor decisions and our memory falters. It ages us prematurely and makes us short-tempered. Stress alters our hormonal balance and metabolism.

We are not machines. We cannot endlessly violate our bodies with tension and emotional maelstroms without a revolt or retaliation. We overwhelm our senses with information, but neglect the sensual requirements of our spirit. Humans have rapidly accepted ridiculous lifestyles filled with multi-tasking, excessive work hours, and performance anxiety. Sometimes we are time pressured by scheduling our days to the minute. We create a larger digital footprint in one day, from debit cards, to Facebook, to reward programs, than our grandparents did during their whole lives. Information rapidly comes in and goes out. Human beings have output more data in the past two years than the last 3000 years[1].

We are steeped in a tremendous amount of stimulus. We are so inundated by various to-dos and tasks that we accommodate the onslaught of data in and data out with the expectation that it will make life easier. Many of us do not realize we need to manage and limit it for the health of our bodies and our minds. We are constantly being monitored by cameras and blitzed with rules, regulations, and fines. Technology has advanced at an astronomical rate, but our bodies were not designed to absorb this at an endless and exponentially increasing pace. If we do not regulate this level of both obvious and insidious stress and if we do not equalize our lives, we set ourselves up for a fall. I suspect this alone can account for a measure in the massive rise of diseases and chronic conditions.

I observe and study people due to my curiosity about their levels of health, happiness, and what they label success. One strong theme I notice frequently is people fostering a complicated life. When you are overtaxing yourself with a convoluted lifestyle, wearing too many hats with too many tasks, tension escalates.

---

1   KSPS: The Human Face of Big Data

We are the creators of our lives. We decide to take on more than is necessary. We agree to put our kids in too many activities. We choose our high-pressure careers. Simplifying our lives is one of the greatest anti-stress strategies we can implement. A simple life is a sweet life.

Cancer is a wake-up call to make a change. In cancer hospitals and with friends diagnosed I have heard over and over again, "I just want to get back to normal."

I beg to differ. Loudly.

Cancer can only proliferate when equilibrium is compromised.

It is a failure of the body's cells to communicate properly. Your body's ecosystem was in some way disrupted in order for cancer to flourish. And something in your lifestyle or inner emotional world may have tipped the scales. If you can be honest with yourself, you will know this to be true.

Recognizing the stress we live in is not an invitation to self-blame. It is about accountability. And the opportunity for liberation. Life has a way of getting us to course-correct. At times we need something as radical as cancer to make alterations to our emotional states, habits, and lifestyle. The purpose behind your cancer is likely far greater than the inconvenience of it. When we acknowledge the message and make the changes it asks of us, cancer can make an exodus.

When I first traversed the territory of cancer at only 29 years of age, I was a giddy newlywed. My husband was supportive and loving through my journey. But with the abrupt halt to our honeymoon phase, I quickly I realized I had—with eyes wide open—married a man who had a completely different idea of what marriage meant than I did. I loved him dearly, but as time passed, I dug deep and asked myself: with whatever time I have left on Earth, do I want to live it under a cloud of anxiety and crazy-making? The painful answer was no. Although I went into my marriage wholeheartedly with the intention of spending a lifetime with my husband, for the sake of my health and happiness, I knew I had to make the gut-wrenching decision to divorce after only three-and-a-half years.

The second time I was diagnosed, I was still on a high from the successful summer launch of my first travel memoir. I had worked my derrière off, but it was a dream come true—I'd finally had the guts to write about my wanton adventures and readers were responding with enthusiasm. However, two traumatic events had occurred in my life that same summer.

The first one was a short-lived romance with an exciting, exotic man who quickly revealed himself to be the most narcissistic and neurotic person I had ever met. The way the relationship unfolded broke something in me. I took his behavior personally and I began to drown in a sea disappointment. I felt that my love life had plunged to the darkest depths of the ocean. I believed I was done with love. For someone who loves love, it had a profoundly negative impact on my emotional life. I gave up on something of tremendous value to me.

Secondly, the Canadian economy took a dive in 2009. Although most businesses were seeing a huge decline in sales, with the strong client relationships I had built, I kept my territory in luxury sales at a mere 6% decline. It was a worthy feat.

But the young, inexperienced managers I worked for saw the economy as an opportunity to cut my wage in half. In doing so, they slashed my self-worth. I will state categorically that I *allowed* myself to feel and be under-valued. The minute I was given that news, everything in me screamed, "QUIT!" Instead of leaving, I sat on the fence, miserable. I awoke every morning dreading the day ahead. I was unhappy about the circumstances of my life, yet paralyzed. Six months later, I found a lump in my other breast.

There are doctors and practitioners who believe cancer can follow on the heels of a traumatic event. I tell these stories to illustrate how shock, trauma, or a harrowing ordeal can impact our bodies, right down to the cells. I allowed myself to indulge in extreme emotions—and to wallow in self-pity—as do many. Admitting with absolute self-honesty where our lives may not be serving our health and wellbeing is an important part of our healing.

In reflection, I am not surprised that after a twenty-year victory, cancer made a return visit. I can see how the latent gene could well have been triggered (see chapter: Epigenetics). How we perceive the events of our lives dictates our stress levels and outcomes. Our perception of the world is monumental.

It is unlikely the doctors you will deal with on your journey will ask you how much nervous energy you carry on a regular basis. We learn to accept this edginess as normal, as the background buzz of our lives, but it is *not* normal for a healthy, happy system.

Do you have an underlying anxiety woven through your body about anything? Are you constantly thinking about debt or perseverating about a relationship issue? Do you always have a feeling that the other shoe is about to drop or, like Chicken Little, that the sky is about to fall? This type of perpetual dread, even if low-grade, erodes the immune system like a slow rusting on steel.

Your body has likely given you warning signals prior to your diagnosis. As I write this book, I am currently experiencing the dissipation of severe headaches. They began a few weeks before Christmas (it is now the end of February) and came on with a vengeance. I have never had headaches like this before; they were exceedingly painful and wreaking havoc with my energy levels.

When I took a vacation, the headaches receded within two days. A few days after returning home, they reappeared just as acutely as before. My doctor gave me a requisition for a brain scan, but I suspected I would find the source of the issue.

Last week, an unpleasant incident occurred with one of my contractual positions; I knew that the only thing to do was resign, effective immediately. In spite of my fears about the financial impact, I did it anyway. The headaches drastically dissipated within days. Our bodies will warn us when the things we do are a disservice to our overall welfare.

Hidden stress can creep up on us in ways we may not acknowledge. If you have given up on a dream, or have a loss of direction or purpose, this can be an underlying source of chronic misery. Self-recrimination for past mistakes, or a constant cloud of guilt or shame, influences our wellbeing. Feelings of being under-appreciated, overlooked, or forgotten wear on our psyche. Deep disappointments in life can haunt us and affect our health.

The most erroneous thing you can do is "get back to normal." Listen to your body and its intuitive nudgings and make no more excuses for overloading yourself with too much work, staying in bad relationships, or consenting to undervaluation. Procrastinating or refusing to deal with the issues that need to be taken care of may have had serious implications.

The good news is, it is reversible and you can choose to courageously and honestly address the changes required for a healthy, wonderful life moving forward.

Lighten Up, Francis!
01/31/2014

"Last night I lost the world, and gained the Universe."
—C. JoyBell C.

When we were young, my sister and I would shout "Lighten Up Francis!" if the other was getting a tad too bitchy. Now later in life, we use the expression when either of us becomes overly gloomy or analytical about an issue in our lives. (I couldn't remember where we got the phrase from, so I did a little research. It's from the movie *Stripes**)

In my twenties, life was a beach. Or rather a beach party. Even though I worked damned hard, I didn't sweat it too much and my main concern was how much fun and play I could squeeze into a day. As I matured, life became much more serious and a lot less light.

Over a decade ago, I created a New Year's tradition that I have since shared with my girlfriends at our annual party. I dedicate an entire evening to authoring and handwriting New Year's wishes for the upcoming year whilst listening to Christmas music. I think about the women I will distribute the wishes to and set the intention that each will get the perfect message they need at that moment, myself included. I sometimes add images from magazines or stickers and I seal each wish in an envelope so that they are a blind and random pick.

This year my envelope held the following:

"For 2014 I wish for you ...

That you completely lighten up! That whatever is heavy or stressful in your life is lifted from your mind and heart and that you feel so light, so joy-filled, and so happy that you dance and sing spontaneously almost every day!"

I squinted as I read my pick. There were certainly many selections in the bag that I could have used; the wishes are varied—they are about health, a soul mate, home, travel, windfalls, career success, hot sex, beauty and fitness, and magic and miracles. But within seconds I laughed and realized that this was the right wish for me.

When we set a goal or have a profound desire for pretty much anything, what is the actual bottom line? If you dig deeper past the obvious (e.g., I want to be a wildly successful author) it's not the *thing*, it's the feeling one receives from the desire: freedom, accomplishment, happiness, security, contentment, bliss, or a sense of making a difference.

For any of my goals or dreams, my core aspiration is to feel like I want to sing *Zip-a-Dee-Doo-Dah*[1] from the rooftops. Preparing for Mexico in December—the place that makes my heart happy—I found myself in occasional bouts of dancing and singing.

Lightening up takes constant vigilance. We can lose sight of it because life has a way of making us forget the joy to be had *if* we were to make joy our first priority.

What obliterates our lightheartedness?

Usually, the past. Or more precisely, thinking about it. Dredging up previous hurts, rejections, perceived failures, criticisms, regrets, fears, slights, losses, or hardships. And remember, the past can be as recent as yesterday.

The cure? Let it go. *Ha ha ha ha ha*! You laugh. We love hanging onto our stories and our pain. But what if we were to just let it go, man? What if we made a decision to release it all into the wind?

My sister and I discussed a personal dilemma this weekend that mirrored her own impasse a couple of months ago. Afterward she brilliantly said, "You've done everything you can, now let it go. No need for more analysis or dissection. Don't destroy it by flogging it. Just let it be whatever it will be. I ruined my own fun by over-analyzing. Don't make the same mistake."

Hmmph. What a novel concept. Don't let it swirl and twirl and catch in the pathways of your brain, don't let it fester and swell into something painful, just let it go.

Sometimes we buy the bull that life is meant to be hard, somber and that we should take ourselves oh so seriously. There is grim pleasure in making a mountain out of a molehill: we can all find the payoff in our juicy tales of woe.

Our ebullience—our singing, or belly cackling, or outright goofiness—far more than our woes—can pose a threat to others. Some may even try to squash us by admonishing that we are being silly or irresponsible.

---

1 https://youtu.be/6bWyhj7siEY

Illegitimi non carborundum. Kind of sounds like a Harry Potter spell, but it roughly means: don't let the bastards grind you down!

Here are a few ideas for lightening up, Francis:

- Actively and doggedly seek humor and laughter.
- Smile more at everyone. Much more.
- Talk to strangers.
- Be crazy generous.
- Truly absorb nature.
- Appreciate, appreciate, appreciate.

P.S. If you can't quite get the concept of letting it go (like me), get Bob Newhart's Life Coaching advice on how to do it. (Hint: it's worth 6 minutes for the giggle.)

https://youtu.be/MDpyS2HN5SA

Bob Newhart 'Stop It'
https://youtu.be/Ow0lr63y4Mw

Lighten up, Francis
http://wp.me/p2ACw4-kA
lifebyheart.wandasthilaire.com

16

Nature

*"There is pleasure in the pathless woods. There is rapture on the lonely shore.
There is society where none intrudes, by the deep sea, and music in its roar: I
love not man the less, but Nature more."*
—Lord Byron

We in the cities have dissociated from the benefits of connecting to the earth. The strain is slow and insidious and we do not realize the negative effects of the steady assault of noise and heavy traffic as we go about our days surrounded by cement.

We rush around on deadlines. We are ruled and regulated to death. 'Big Brother' watches us with cameras on every corner tracking our speed and vigilantly monitoring our parking meters. We are inundated with emails and expectations. We spend inordinate amounts of time in front of computers and televisions. We have become steeped in a fight-or-flight lifestyle, constantly filtering data, danger, and distractions. There is nothing healthy or natural about any of this and it messes with our inner ecosystem.

A divine pulse permeates the natural realm, one that realigns our internal rhythms. Nature is based on cooperation, not competition and a fundamental harmony is weaved within it. If there is anything I have come to learn from the master teacher, cancer, it is the preciousness and holiness of nature.

When you sit and truly observe the natural environment—when you fully absorb it—you enter a whole new world of awesomeness. It is one of the most soothing things you can do for yourself. It literally calms down the part of the brain that has been overtaxed, which in turn helps to bring the body into coherence.

The Japanese have a term for spending time in nature called *shin-rin-yoku* (forest bathing). It is the act of taking therapeutic visitations in a forest for rejuvenation where the trees and foliage give off beneficial and medicinal scents and good bacteria.

I was once given a stargazing assignment.

For the next five nights in a row, we ask that you find a place where you have an excellent view of the night sky. You may even want to drive to a hill so that the celestial panorama is even more visible. Prepare yourself with the correct clothing to be outdoors so that you are very comfortable and not distracted by the chill.

And then sit and watch the sky.

When you feel antsy or tempted to get back indoors, or into the car, sit some more. Allow your mind to wander amongst the stars; visit the galaxies and dance with the cosmic music that you will begin to hear. You may wish to journal your experiences and if the impetus is there, follow it. This will take you from doing to being. (I outline the results of this assignment in the blog post *To Be or Not To Be* on page 167. *Permission, Terry Kohl.*)

Heading into a harsh Canadian winter after treatment, my heart told me that I needed nature and sunshine for my healing. I knew that I could not return to my career or my old life as it had been, and my new beginning started in nature. I would be turning 50 and the appearance of cancer was not the way I had envisioned ringing in such a significant year. I had no desire for a big party. I wanted to celebrate by doing what I love most—being on the ocean surrounded by sea life with a few friends and family. I put out the intention to see whales, dolphins, manta rays, and a turtle. Mother Nature came through and gave me all of them.

Many years earlier I discovered nature's value and healing power. After a whirlwind romance, I left France dejected, suffering from the most monumental heartbreak of my life. My original plan for a six-month stay in France was turned upside down swiftly and I subsequently decided that the best place to recover from my broken heart and shattered life would be Mexico. I shudder to think of what would have happened had I turned around and gone back to Canada in the dead of wintertime.

In Mexico, the sea, the sand, the sun, and the marine life all helped to mend my devastated spirit.

Sunlight is therapy and it feeds the body. We are now heavily indoctrinated to stay out of the sun because of skin cancer, but we need vitamin D, especially people who have had cancer. I am fair-skinned, but I almost never burn because I use common sense and I don't sit and sun bake on the beach. I use sunscreen, but not 75. The right kind of sunscreen blocks UVA, but does not block UVB.

I have traveled for sales most of my life. When I was assigned to visit rural locations, I equipped my car with a deluxe folding chair, books, water, and snacks. In the summer months after a long day of calls, I would drive back to the city via the back roads and choose a serene spot to situate myself. I live near the Rockies, so sometimes I would pick a place with a stunning mountain vista. Other times I sat near a pond. And occasionally, I would sit right in the middle of a wheat field. Many a curious cowboy stopped to ask what I was doing. They would all scratch their heads when I told them I was on a nature break from the city. I found it a phenomenal way to de-stress.

If you already live on a farm or in nature, you are at a major advantage. If you have been dashing past life in the city, observe the natural world now with slow sensuality. This is what really matters. Be excited by the tiniest wonders of the world, right here and now. Take a walk. Look at the flowers and watch the birds as they build their nests and dart about. Lie on the grass and cloud gaze. Lean against a big, beautiful tree and read a book. Watch the sun as it sets and the moon as it rises. Sit near running water such as a brook or waterfall, a fountain or waves. Rain and flowing water release negative ions (negative in this case meaning a good thing for wellbeing). Nature is, in a manner of speaking, designed to speed our recovery and boost our resilience to the stresses of life and the trials of illness.

Time spent in nature always clears my head and graces me with a new perspective. I went to the mountains while writing this chapter and as I walked through the trees along a stream, I had an epiphany with a brilliant solution to a problem that presented itself like a movie in my mind.

Life existed for millennia with human beings working in harmony and peaceful co-existence with Earth. We followed the rhythms of nature and used plants to heal our ailments. We worked with the meridian energy (chi) in the body to rebalance our systems. It is only since the Information Age that we abandoned ancient wisdom and forgot that our bodies were created in synchronization with the planet in a non-toxic, non-harmful coherence.

The tremendous beauty and geometric wonders of nature freely and abundantly offers our minds and bodies a sacred space for healing, peace, and pure joy. The interconnectedness of life will reveal itself if you stop to observe it.

Nature has answers.
Nature heals.

The Lost Art
7/31/2016

As I travel alone
on unplanned adventures
sitting
observing
breathtaking scenes etched eternally in my memory
when the notion of time is elusive
the gypsy in my soul
tells me home is anywhere I am
—Wanda St. Hilaire
Of Love, Life and Journeys

Last night, a friend and I went to watch an outdoor performance by some surprisingly talented young singers. Minutes after a lone songstress began to play in the gazebo, a rain shower hit. I was impressed to see most of the adults pull out their umbrellas rather than scatter. A large group of children played in a patch of grass and not a single one flinched at the rain. They danced and twirled and carried on with their games. The little ones were a reminder of the freedom we can have when we let go of our hang-ups and fixations on how things must be.

When the rain stopped, we were gifted with an idyllic summer evening. Scads of sailboats dotted the water and on a walk along the wooded reservoir we had a spectacular view of the mountains as the sun descended.

When we came around a bend, we saw a mesmerized mob of people loitering and staring at their cellphones. I had heard of, but not seen, the Pokémon lunacy until then. Like lemmings heading over a cliff, more phone-toting fools were making their way to this port of addiction. We were in an oasis of nature in the middle of the city on a rare, perfect night and the only thing these people were interested in was an inane game on a small electronic device.

Any master—be they artist, writer, photographer, dancer, or scientist—has cultivated the art of observation. It is the way we make the necessary connections for creativity and the how of tapping into our genius. Our great poets are and were observers extraordinaire. Walt Whitman and Ralph Waldo Emerson found inspiration in bearing witness to nature and spending hours in quiet reflection.

To catch the unusual or the unexpected in science and research, honed habits of observation are more important than education. Wilfred Trotter, the godfather of neuroscience said, *"Knowledge comes from noticing resemblances and recurrences in the events that happen around us."*

In medicine, any good healer or doctor should have a keen sense of observation and not rely solely on tests and diagnostics. If we listen to and observe our own bodies they will tell us what we need or what is out of balance. One night I said a small prayer for my health. In the morning I awakened saying the word "lycopene" aloud. This is a powerhouse antioxidant, so I immediately went out to purchase a bottle and ate two large lycopene-rich watermelons and a batch of tomatoes over the next few weeks. I assumed my body had told me clearly (and weirdly) what it needed.

I once read a National Geographic article about acclaimed nature photographers who were octogenarians and some even nonagenarians. These men and women had spent their lives observing the natural world. In order to capture beauty, they immersed themselves in textures, tones, and the many hues of light. They were happy and still highly productive. Seeking the rare and the majestic, they were insulated from depression and anxiety. Observing, walking, and creating works of art kept them mentally sharp and physically well. They derived great satisfaction and a sense of purpose from photography, and none had retired.

On another gorgeous summer day after our torrential rains, I meandered along my favorite river path. Every single man on a bicycle whizzed past me as fast as they could go and each one had a stern look as though they had to get somewhere very, very important. I'm betting not. No smiling. No catching the beauty.

A snake tangled up on a rock sunning itself caught my eye. I jumped with a start and then stopped to observe it. My fear of snakes is second only to my arachnophobia, but I felt this creature deserved some acknowledgment. In many cultures, the snake is revered as a symbol of life and positive transitions. He sat flicking his forked tongue and decided to slither around and then take refuge under the rock. Slithering is the part that scares me most and I forced myself to stay put and watch. Observing the snake, rather than fleeing, I left him less frightened than I have ever been.

Consciously going out into nature with the intention of witnessing and being fully present, I find treasures and wonders on my walks. I have taught myself to look for specific things that hold significance for me. It requires a development of pattern recognition, of training the eye to notice one small thing that doesn't belong. I find feathers, coins, trinkets, pertinent messages on paper, and even photos. On my suburban walk on the Canyon Meadow ridge I have seen black hawks circling, a pheasant on a rooftop, white-tailed deer grazing, many rabbits scampering, and have heard coyotes howling at sunset. I seek the unusual and the beautiful.

In order to write and be a storyteller, I must observe. Even though I am a social creature, this is one of the reasons I enjoy solo travel. When I am alone, my detection skills are heightened by leaps and bounds. I see things I would never notice if I were distracted by another. I hear things I may not catch if I were in a constant dialogue. And I love the immersion into a new place when my attention is fully on the moment.

When faced with a problem or condition, we get a new perspective if we can step away from ourselves (and any confusion or anxiety) and observe the situation as a bystander would. Like Sherlock Holmes, we can see pieces of our personal puzzle that begin to connect and fit. We may make new deductions as we unearth information.

One of the most valuable gifts in the art of observation lies in its side effect: it removes our blinders and prompts us to notice things we had previously missed. There is infinitely more in our world than what we perceive as we dash around, only because we have not consciously cultivated the ability to see things we do not understand—things that are not rational and that we have no previous frame of reference for. When we only look for the expected, that is what we will find.

Years ago, I went to a launch for a photo book called *Seeing Evangeline*[1], which was filled with plants and flowers in various stages of decline and decay that looked like fairies. The photographer exposed the most amazing faces and creatures hidden within nature and it was

---

1   http://seeingevangeline.com/

truly magical. Her work reminds her readers to use their imaginations and actively hunt for the mystical.

If you have any interest in spotting the supernatural—actively look for it. If you would like to see things you did not know existed, open your eyes with a different lens, one that engages all of your senses, including your sixth. Ask your heart to lead you away from the commonplace and into the enchantment that still exists on this, our planet Earth.

The Lost Art
http://wp.me/p2ACw4-zr
lifebyheart.wandasthilaire.com

17

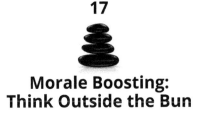

Morale Boosting:
Think Outside the Bun

"Freedom began on the day the first sheep wandered away from the herd."
—Marty Rubin

Most of the cancer cog is morose. Where I live, everything is done in an institutional setting. Hospitals and cancer treatment centers are full of hyper serious people and it can be emotionally exhausting. If you buy into the somber silence in the halls and waiting rooms, you could find yourself sucked into a pit of sorrow. I highly recommend you create your own reality going through cancer.

During my first stint, I was kept in the hospital for a week. That was when nurses in Canada were still given the time to actually nurse. Breast cancer at 29 was rare in 1990, and someone—nobody knows who—gave me a private room in a corner, likely because of the high volume of visitors. I had no restrictions and the nurses allowed my friends to come and go all hours of the day and night.

A newlywed, I brought with me photos of our wedding and honeymoon. I had special mementos from home in my room as well. I took a pretty robe and slippers and wore make-up to feel better.

When I went in for surgery, I asked the surgical team not to speak negatively about my situation in the operating room. I did not want to subconsciously pick up ideas of a poor outcome.

The second time in radiation I made sure to engage the technicians. For my first treatment I had my sister write *'Hello!'* on my right breast and on my last day write *'Gracias and Good-bye!'* I made sure these women knew I was a human being and not just another body to irradiate. We talked about my travels and my book, *The Cuban Chronicles*, and I gave them advice on traveling solo. I quipped and kept my sense of humor, which was, I surmised, a bit of a reprieve from the sadness they see each day.

At my afternoon treatments, a Caribbean couple sat in the waiting area at the same time. My sister accompanied me to all appointments and we befriended Ben and Julianne. We would laugh and swap stories. Sometimes the techs would poke their heads out of their office to see what was going on because laughter was uncommon.

My sister brought them fresh Okanagan fruit; they brought us home-grown potatoes and Jamaican patties. After our coinciding last treatment, we brought a candle-laden pie inscribed with 'Yippee!' and a bottle of açaí berry juice for a toast. We sang, 'Happy Health Day to Us,' took pictures, and hooted in celebration outside the cancer center at a picnic table.

Morale boosting ideas ...

- For doctor's appointments and treatments bring a headset and listen to whatever music makes you feel good. There are thousands of calming hypnosis downloads with ocean sounds or tranquil music available.

- Take small travel breaks if that feeds your soul. Go away between treatments for a refreshing change of scenery if you can. Should you have friends or family with a cottage or getaway home, ask if they would be willing to let you stay for a short time. Use up your travel points or buddy passes. My friend has been going through chemotherapy once again and still goes away with her husband to see their beloved Red Sox for an injection of fun into her life during a difficult time. They made a one-month trip to Mexico and she made arrangements for her required blood transfusion at the local hospital.

- If you want to take complementary treatments, know that it need not be a ridiculously expensive venture. I stayed at an economical apartment in Mexico on a per month basis during alternative treatments. I ate organically and visited juice stands that offered healthy smoothies and green drinks each day at a fraction of the cost in Canada. The juice vendor asked me what I was doing in Vallarta; he suspected I was not on a vacation. He wrote out a healing recipe specifically for cancer and when I did not have time to search for the ingredients, he went shopping for the special combination of items—and gifted them to me.

- Poetry is food for the soul. You may never have taken the time to discover it, but it could be something to soothe you right now. You can pick up the classics at a public library or find poetry books at your local Goodwill.

• For $5+ you can have a personalized mind movie made of your healthy and happy life. It is a powerfully uplifting visual medley with music, images, and captions of your choice. I had one made on fiverr. com (if you want to see examples, do a "mind movies" search on YouTube). Watch it on a daily basis to imprint your imagination with wellness.

• During the second episode I had two radiation treatments per day. I booked an appointment with a Body Talk energy healer at the end of each day to help clear my system of excess radiation and to boost my energy. I don't know if it was the placebo effect or if it genuinely offset the effects of the radiation, but it helped.

• Get advice on the best choice of oils and buy an infuser from a quality essential oil shop. Keep it in your bedroom, meditation, or reading room. Essential oils are healing and have a positive impact on mood.

• If you are able to focus, indulge in frivolous or epic novels. Get unusual magazines to peruse if your attention span is short right now. Follow blogs that are about subjects you love.

• Find vlogs (video blogs) on YouTube with vloggers whose content resonates.

• Have lots of unstructured, spontaneous "play" and down time.

• Buy a box of sidewalk chalk and draw or write messages along your favorite path—things like 'You are loved' 'You are beautiful' 'Follow your bliss' and 'You are amazing.' It will make someone's day—guaranteed.

• Simplify your life to the most minimal of obligations, chores, and drudgery.

• If you have a partner, stay sexually active in some capacity.

- Send yourself uplifting postcards in the mail.

- If you don't have pets, borrow someone's dog or cat to bond with and cuddle or spend some time on a farm.

- Watch children play in a park.

- Let people hug you.

Denmark is rated as one of the happiest countries in the world. The Danes have a cultural term called hygge (pronounced 'hooga'), which is a part of the happiness factor, in spite of long, cold winters with short days. The word is imbued with coziness and simple pleasure. It is derived from a Norwegian word meaning wellbeing. Hygge is an abstract concept with broad meaning; one that translator ToveMaren Stakkestad said was never meant to be translated, but rather to be felt.

Hygge appears to be the art of creating a well-lived life. It is deep contentment found through a sense of togetherness and belonging. It's camaraderie; sharing hearty meals with friends or lingering around a fireplace with mulled cider. It's crafting a relaxing atmosphere with candlelight, charm, and beauty.

In solitude, it's rituals like reading a book snuggled under a thick duvet with a hot tea and writing in a gratitude journal over a latte. It's indulging in cozy PJs and slippers. It's building a sanctuary of serenity and being kind to yourself.

Hygge is an attitude based on the idea of overall wellness—weaving spirit into the daily grind and making the ordinary enchanted. It is something we would be well served by to borrow from the Danes.

Use your imagination. Think of alternatives to the bleak road well-travelled. Awaken people along the way and surprise them. You do not have to follow the masses down the trail of misery. It is your unique journey—exert control over it by the choices you make and keep your morale high by doing things you know will feed your soul.

18

Fill Your Mind With Possibility

"Become a possibilitarian. No matter how dark things seem to be or actually are, raise your sights and see possibilities—always see them for they are always there."
—Norman Vincent Peale

My all-time favorite cancer survival story is of a Greek man named Stamis Moraitis. Stamis had immigrated to the USA and landed a job doing manual labor. He married a Greek-American woman and later moved to Florida.

One day in his mid-sixties, he became short of breath. Tests revealed lung cancer. He sought many opinions and the doctors gave him nine months to live. An aggressive treatment regime was recommended, but upon reflection, he decided to return to Ikaria, Greece where he could be buried with his family overlooking the Aegean Sea.

He and his wife moved in with his elderly parents at their tiny, picturesque vineyard. He was bedridden most of the time when he first arrived. Old friends began filing over for lingering visits, as Greeks do, with a bottle of wine and fresh food. On Sunday mornings he tottered to the church he had known as a child, reconnecting with his faith.

He began to feel stronger, so he planted a garden for his wife in the sunshine and ocean air of the Greek island. He lived to harvest it and started working in the vineyard, reacquainting himself with a sweet and sensuous Mediterranean lifestyle.

In 2013, thirty-six years after his diagnosis, without surgery, radiation, or chemotherapy, he died at the age of 98.

I have been to the Greek Islands and I know why he healed. Life is slow and rich there. The wine is organically produced and the food goes from picking to table. The renowned Mediterranean diet, rich in omega oil, is health affirming. The sense of community is astoundingly strong.

I was on the island of Mykonos for a week when I moved *pensiones* one afternoon. As I stood at the cash machine near the pier, I fretted. I had to pay for my room, but discovered that the only two terminals on the island were down late on a Friday afternoon and the landlady would not give me my passport or luggage until I paid.

At that point, it seemed as though everyone on the island knew who I was. A nearby waiter noticed and came over to ask what was wrong. After I explained, he pulled a wad of cash from his apron and offered it to me. I was surprised considering the number of foreigners coming and going and declined his generous offer of a loan, thinking I would find a solution.

I hiked through the town's maze to a sunglass shop where I had made a purchase to test my card for a malfunction. It worked fine. The owner was apologetic that he had no cash to loan me.

Next, I sat on the patio at a cappuccino bar I had been frequenting to ponder the situation. The owner noticed my consternation and asked me what had happened. Again, I explained. He pulled a bundle of cash from his pocket and gave it to me.

"Pay me back when the bank machine is fixed."

Later that evening, I was sipping a glass of iced ouzo in a little bar where I'd had dinner when the sunglass shopkeeper ran up to me out of breath. He plopped a handful of drachmas down in front of me.

"I was so worried about you! Here is the money for the *pensione*."

I was speechless. After only a week on that little Greek island, the locals were watching out for me with tremendous love that still lives in my heart.

When you are in a culture of support and community, as was Stamis, you are in a place that inspires healing.

The well-documented story Anita Moorjani shares in her book, *Dying to be Me*, is another miraculous tale that moved me to the core. Moorjani was rushed to a hospital in Singapore where she fell into a coma. She was in the final stages of lymphoma, her body covered in lemon-sized tumors and her organs failing. The senior oncologist told her husband she would not survive past 36 hours and they prepared a medication drip to ease her passage.

She drifted into a near death experience where she had an epiphany about the purpose of her cancer and how she had gotten that far along into the illness. When she awoke, the doctors warned her family it was temporary and that death was imminent. But to the surprise of everyone, she came out the coma and rapidly began healing. After knocking at death's doorstep, she is alive and well, telling her tale of triumph and sharing the wisdom she derived from her cancer journey and miraculous healing (which was medically verified and extensively documented). Her journey is one of tremendous hope for cancer patients, one I highly recommend reading.

There are many people alive today who have beaten "incurable" and "terminal" cancer. Miracles do not fit into the medical model, so you are not likely to find mention of them in a hospital or a doctor's office. But the stories abound. You can find them in books and on the Internet. *Chicken Soup for the Soul* is chock-full of stories of victory. Keep your eyes on them. Fill your mind with them. Water and feed your desire to manifest them.

The cool thing about planet Earth is that *impossible things happen every day.*

Believe it.

TEDxBayArea | Dying to be me!
Anita Moorjani
https://youtu.be/rhcJNJbRJ6U
http://www.anitamoorjani.com

The Art of Impossibility

> *"I would never die for my beliefs because I might be wrong."*
> —Bertrand Russell

Did you know that the delectable and delicious tomato was once believed to be a deadly poisonous nightshade and was even associated with witchcraft? And that in Papua New Guinea, some tribes believed babies were made bit by bit with repeated—as often as a man could manage—intercourse? (Okay, not such a bad belief ...)

At an intimate celebration with a delightful artist couple I know, I told them of a neurotic boyfriend I once had for a wee time who wore a hoodie to bed in July in +30 degree weather. He believed that if he caught the slightest breeze, he would fall ill and die because he had a minor (I'm guessing imaginary) throat tickle.

My friend blanched and confessed she too wore a hoodie to bed. What!? She is from (the former) Yugoslavia and she told me how she was cautioned her whole life to avoid drafts at all costs. If she was caught sitting on the ground, her aunts would scream at her to get up, because she would surely be barren and have health issues due to the cold earth. She is always careful to cover her hip area and wears massive amounts of neck and headgear in winter. Her culture has even devised a specially knit "skirt" to protect a woman's womb and grooms often gift these to brides instead of lingerie.

I asked what her mother and her aunts would think of my 365-day-a-year habit of sleeping nude with a window wide open and sometimes with a fan blowing directly on my skin. She was visibly mortified. It would be akin to medical heresy and almost certain death.

Human belief is a subject that absolutely fascinates me. I am a seeker of the secret to permanently changing dysfunctional beliefs—the kind that hold people back from living their biggest and best life. Many experts in psychology and human behavior state that our beliefs create the outcome of our lives *implicitly*. As an example, my friend above now has recurring kidney and bladder troubles.

A new friend of mine is a life coach and we have had deep discussions on the immense power of our beliefs. We hear old adages like "Whatever the mind can conceive and believe, it can achieve" (Napoleon Hill) and think *ya, ya*. That's okay for those guys, but I'm too old or too broke or too tired or have too many responsibilities to dream. I don't have a degree, or the talent, or the looks.

We are surrounded by 'impossible' things that are now reality: Google Earth; iPhones; bionic limbs; and electric cars. Big thinkers do not let obstacles or small thinking get in their way to achieving incredible things. And you can bet that when something doesn't work for the innovators of the world, they change their strategy. They transcend their doubt, and in spite of the blood, sweat, tears, and Herculean effort involved, they just do it.

For me, the past often pulls and tugs at my dreams, dragging them down into the murky land of impossibility. There are many recollections of falls that are tattooed into my brain. *Alert! Alert! Remember! ... The last time you did that, look what happened.*

Think about some of the things you would like to do, be, or have. Consider things you have tucked away on a dusty shelf somewhere in the recesses of your mind because they seemed impossible. Then watch Aussie Nick Vujicic in action: Life Without Limbs: Nick Vujicic—Never Give Up[1].

Nick was born with a rare disorder that left him limbless. It seems like one of the biggest hurdles a human being could face. Nick had his share of struggles and emotional turmoil as a child and contemplated suicide at age ten, but at seventeen founded a non-profit organization called *Life Without Limbs*[2].

Nick began a career as a motivational speaker. In polls, our fear of public speaking outranks our fear of death because we are terrified of public ridicule and of looking foolish. We worry about being judged for our weight or our appearance. Imagine finding the courage to speak to massive audiences when you are *limbless*.

Nick has adapted beyond what anyone could have imagined. He has two toes that he writes, uses the computer, and cooks with. He swims (yes, swims), plays golf, soccer, and has skydived.

I have moments when I feel there must be something fundamentally

---

1   https://youtu.be/kD-fH5W_Ruk
2   http://www.lifewithoutlimbs.org/

wrong with me to remain single for so long and that finding love is an illusive fantasy. Nick dreamed of meeting the love of his life and then met a stunning girl named Kanae Miyahara and married her[1] in February of 2012. This February, one day before Valentine's Day, they had a healthy baby boy.

Now reach into your mind's eye again and consider some physical feat you have imagined yourself doing, but have decided is absolutely unachievable. Then ponder the scientifically "impossible" achievement of Diana Nyad.

On September 19th of this year, 64-year old Nyad set a world record by swimming from Cuba[2] to Florida's coastline—without a shark cage—an unprecedented feat.

It was her fifth attempt and she had not swam for 30 years when she began training at age 60. On her third attempt, she was bitten by the deadly box jellyfish and began to go into respiratory shock. That alone would be enough to send the toughest packing.

I listened to Nyad eloquently speak this week on Oprah's part one of the interview. The preparation that is involved and the team of experts required to attempt such a swim are mind-boggling.

The things that happen to a human body when immersed in salt water for such an extended period of time (53 hours) while employing that much physical energy is utterly frightening. Physiologists determined that, by all of their calculations, based on her age and all statistics on the navigational data, it could not be done.

Nyad emerged from the water severely dehydrated and looked like a beat up blowfish, yet less than 72 hours later she was laughing and powerfully orating her tale at a press conference.

What medicine and science is unable to measure is the human spirit and will. It has gone awry countless times when predicting when someone will die of an "incurable" disease or what a human being is capable of achieving. There is a force we all have access to that defies logic.

Diana Nyad achieved the impossible at age 64 because she *believed* she could. Nick Vujicic changed his perspective and decided that he could create a full, bountiful life in spite of seemingly insurmountable odds

1 https://youtu.be/3Ux5TMfhCgY
2 https://youtu.be/jt1WeDq-rZc

against it and he is living that big, bold life, with hundreds of thousands of fans in his wake.

We love stories of amazing achievements and wildly impossible happenstances, but in our own lives we have a tendency to place a tight cap on what is possible. Often, we make projections about the work involved to attain something and decide in advance that we do not have what it takes.

I can't wait to read the new release, *David And Goliath: Underdogs, Misfits, and the Art of Battling Giants*[1], by one of my favorite authors, Malcolm Gladwell. In it he shares stories of ordinary people who have achieved extraordinary things. He too is fascinated with discovering what lies beyond the studied and proven "facts" about the human capacity.

I still do not know why some people are able to shed their doubt and rise above their limitations with such grace while others of us are ambushed by our fatigued misgivings.

What I do know is, never underestimate yourself. Inside of you is a reservoir of astonishing ability and endurance that just needs to be released from the rigid cement of disbelief.

I leave you with a poem I wrote at a difficult moment when I needed to access that well within.

A formidable courage resides inside you
The path to your dreams is sometimes treacherous
But cast aside the shroud of skepticism
Ask your imagination for the stepping stones to your aspirations
You have but one fleeting moment here with two choices:

The dark imprisonment of I can't

Or

The enchantment of ...

I can.

—*Wanda St. Hilaire*
Of Love, Life and Journeys

---

1 https://www.amazon.com/gp/0316204366

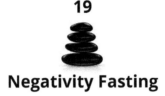

19

Negativity Fasting

Beautiful things happen when you distance yourself from negativity.
—Miss Lucky Sunshine

The medical doctor I conferred with in Mexico wanted to know about my emotional state—in great detail. He asked about my feelings in regard to different facets of my life. He inquired about any recent traumas that had occurred.

The doctor advised me not to be a confidante for anyone's problems or a sounding board for complaining. He suggested that it was best to spend time with friends in uplifting conversations and playtime. I am the kind of person people come to with their problems and I love to help solve them, so it was hard for me to set boundaries. But I did.

You may have people in your life who are chronic complainers or are in a constant state of melodrama and it is perfectly okay for you tell them that you have been prescribed a plan of "positivity." Now is not the time to waste your precious energy on gossip or family squabbles. Stay away from people who drain your energy.

The doctor also asked what type of TV shows and movies I liked to watch and recommended I avoid all heavy drama or violent content while I healed—only funny, romantic, or educational shows. That advice proved to be excellent. It kept me in a more optimistic state of mind.

You may feel that staying informed about the world's affairs is important, but can the bad news wait? Can you take a break from the toxicity of the media? Learning about yet another oil spill or what ISIS is up to will not elevate your mood. The world is increasingly absurd and now is not the time to overwhelm yourself with the insanity. News is systematically designed to scare and shock people and it feeds pessimism. If you are prone to carping about the state of the world, let it be. This is not the time to worry over things you can do nothing about.

If you are overwhelmed with social media and you tend to feel bad after looking at everyone's Facebook posts with pictures of their trips to Tuscany or reading how blissful their lives are (sometimes fantasy), stop scrolling. A lot of what is posted is on social media sites is inane and pointless. The virtual world will wait.

Reality TV will suck the life force out of you. You do not need to focus on the ridiculous problems of people you do not even know. Even though it seems like entertainment, it typically has a negative influence on your mind.

Take a fast from violence. If you fill your mind with gore and killing you will unquestionably deplete your optimism. Watching violent TV and movies is a proven depressant.

David Attenborough's *Planet Earth* series is gorgeous and uplifting. PBS hosts events with thought leaders like Deepak Chopra and Wayne Dyer. BBS has hilarious content like *Mrs. Brown's Boys*. Visit Louie Schwartzberg's YouTube channel[1] to see the wonders of nature with his spectacular photography. Streaming is now available from Gaia TV[2] with fascinating content. For cool documentaries about the nature of the world try Curiosity Stream[3]. Watch children's movies such as *Finding Nemo, Shark Tales*, or *Moana* (the messages in *Moana* are moving). There are so many options for uplifting content. Avoid filling your mind with trash and the suffering of others, even if it is fictitious.

We are assaulted with ads on the Internet, which have an adverse influence on us. I discovered a brilliant ad-blocking program at www.intently.com (both free and upgraded). You handpick the images of health, happiness, family, travel, quotes—whatever you wish to see. Instead of being barraged with ads that have been data targeted to you, the images you see will be appealing and inspiring. It is a valuable application that reduces the inundation of advertising from your life. The best part of Intently is that it blocks irritating ads that run on YouTube. If you do not have the energy, ask someone to set it up for you. It's very simple.

Humor and laughter are potent medicine. They are sustenance for the spirit. In the book *Anatomy of an Illness*, Norman Cousins outlines how he healed himself from a diagnosis of incurable ankylosing spondylitis by taking mega doses of intravenous vitamin C and putting himself on a diet of funny movies and TV programs for many hours each day. He stated that

1 http://tinyurl.com/aeclojp
2 https://www.gaia.com
3 https://www.curiositystream.com/

ten minutes of genuine belly laughing had a two-hour anesthetic effect. No matter what stage you are at with your cancer journey, remember that we all need a good laugh. It lightens the load.

For starters, here is my all-time favorite laugh out loud, tears-running-down-your-face story to get you on your way to the healing power of laughter. It sounds a bit crude, but it's hilarious. (Women tend to find it funnier than men because we fully relate to the mortification factor.) *The Fart that Almost Altered my Destiny*[1]

I never understood the idea of parallel realities until recently. All we need do is observe the people we know to see how each one of them lives a completely different existence. Some choose drama. Some choose adventure. Some choose love. Others choose suffering.

Where we focus our attention is our choice. It is extremely easy to turn life into hell on Earth when we focus on the negativity—of which there is far too much—instead of the sweetness. Cancer is a good time to filter out the ugliness and bring in as much beauty and "positivity" as you can find.

I have created a 'Positivity Playlist' of music on YouTube for your pleasure:
http://tinyurl.com/z6htyjh
(Any ads on playlists listed in this book are not mine.)

1   http://hahasforhoohas.com/the-fart-that-almost-altered-my-destiny

20

Why Me?

I know not why or where they come from
these excruciating physical maladies

From my inner torment?
Grief from unrequited loves?
Bruises to my naïve heart?
Injustices my consciousness or unconsciousness cannot accept?
Or is it solely my divine fate agreed upon before my conception for my time
on Earth?
—Wanda St. Hilaire
Of Love, Life and Journeys

Bad things do happen to good people. I am guessing that *"why me?"* is the burning question of every cancer patient. I live a life of moderation. At 49 I was in the best shape of my life after finding the perfect type of exercise that kept me motivated and happy (Latin dance aerobics).

This is an entry from my journal while getting treatments in Mexico:

My hand hurts under this little cotton ball and bandage where I have had a long needle in my arm for chelation today. While the people on the beach surrounding me are carefree, laughing, and planning frivolous things, I'm thinking about my breast being cut into when I return home.

I see good food everywhere. I'm hungry no matter what I eat. I feel like a vegetarian lizard while people are drinking like fish, eating mountains of greasy food, smoking cigarette after cigarette and roasting in the sun like baked turds—and I am the one with cancer, I am the one eating reptilian fare. I've kept myself healthy, I exercise and I'm in prime shape, I rarely drink, I don't smoke, I eat balanced meals. Today, I don't feel like embracing this shite.

I wholly comprehend the "why me?" conundrum.

A colleague from my past was diagnosed with a wicked type of cancer in which the treatments were disfiguring and painful. She spun her life upside down and backwards trying to figure out why she had this particular type of cancer. You can drive yourself mad with this question. You can spend hours, days, and the rest of your life dissecting your sins. You will, however, never solve anything through analysis of your 'wrongs' and self-torturous obsessing.

When I discovered I had cancer a second time, I was pissed with God, and thoughts of divine retribution welled up inside of me like hot lava. I am not religious, but was brought up Catholic. In my rational adult mind, I knew I was not being punished, but when I was pushed to the brink through the experience, I fell back on my child-self who was indoctrinated with a punitive God.

If you have any notion that you are being punished, let it go. Believe in the loving and unbiased nature of God, the Universe, The Field, or whatever you believe in. For your own peace of mind, know that nothing and no one is meting cruel and unjust punishment on you for some wrongdoing.

Once again, let me remind you that cancer is an imbalance that needs to be addressed. If you are willing to be honest with yourself, you can make changes that will aid and abet your healing. You are not wrong for the decisions you've made. We all do things that help us cope. We make choices that are based on our survival or our sanity. We may use substances that soothe and appease us. Such is the nature of humanity; you are far from alone. Self-blame will only serve to sink your spirits and can take you into a spiral of denial. Reframe harsh self-recrimination into the gentleness of realizing we all do what we do for reasons we consider valid at the time.

There are many better questions to ask yourself than the pointless circular trail of "*why me?*" If you dig deep within and ask the question of your soul from a different slant, "Why am I ill right now?" you will find the answers and be directed to the path of healing.

The Worst Best Things in Life
12/30/2013

"And she thought then how strange it was that disaster—the sort of disaster that drained the blood from your body and took the air out of your lungs and hit you again and again in the face—could be at times, such a thing of beauty."
—Anita Shreve
The Pilot's Wife

Shit happens. And when it does, we ask ourselves, *why is this happening to me? Why now?*

However, if we can move from feeling victimized to uncompromising honesty, we can usually find the message or raison d'être in any colossal event.

In the summer of 1990, I was a ten-month in, giddy-in-love newlywed who was diagnosed with cancer. For a fun-loving, wildly energetic girl at the top of her game, it was like being hit by a semi. As a child, I had watched an aunt die slowly from breast cancer and I thought it was just about the worst thing that could happen to anyone. Now I had it. My husband's love and support greatly helped me through the ordeal and I optimistically jumped each hurdle.

But because of the diagnosis, I realized early into the marriage that in spite of our compatibility and my deep love for this man, his drinking would be the death of me. He was always happy and in a good mood (I suspected—and later learned he had a predilection to stray while under the influence), so I know I would have stayed for many pointless and pain-filled years had I not been given the "life is short" wake-up call. We ended the relationship amicably and I became crystal clear on my values. Travel trumped the list and I vowed I would visit as much of magnificent planet Earth as possible.

When I was dumped in France a few years later by a charming Frenchman I had fallen madly in love with in Portugal, I was devastated well beyond the cancer and the divorce. I had given up my life in Canada to test the waters with this man, but things went south in a heartbeat.

However, that which did not kill me made me stronger. The pain broke open a cascade of words. I began to write and the poetry inspired by that heartbreak became a book, which became a bestseller (by Canadian standards).

I had thought the only reason I could justify to family, friends, or myself, or have the inner strength to move to another country—which I deeply desired—was either for love or career. I discovered that in the worst emotional state of my life, I could not only survive, but also thrive in a foreign country and I made some wonderful friends who are still with me today.

Once past the critical heartbreak phase, I took Spanish lessons and art classes. I designed sundresses and had them sewn for me on the cheap. I flirted boldly with sexy Italian men. I transformed from the despair of thinking I had lost everything to a very bearable lightness of being.

When the Big C returned twenty years later, my work contract was cancelled directly after the diagnosis due to the time off I required. It felt like a monumental double whammy—at first.

But as time went on, I realized I was completely burned out. I dreaded getting up in the mornings and my job felt meaningless. I had proven myself over and over throughout the years with nominal benediction, and I was done. Cutting the cords, albeit cruelly, was just what I needed for my health and wellbeing.

I had not heeded the many signs and messages pre-cancer and it greatly stressed my body. I do believe that the gene that lay benignly in waiting was signaled out of dormancy due to the tension and anxiety I allowed to run amok.

Recently I was hit by the epic Calgary flood. This time the divine message did not take months, weeks, or even days to sink in. Knee deep in mud, digging through my destroyed and drenched belongings, a calm enveloped me and I knew that for me, this event had to happen.

Many times in the previous few years, I had told myself it was time to leave the home I was so profoundly wedged into. But time would slip by with no urgency at hand and my list of things to sort, give up, and pack was left to languish on the fridge.

I knew instantaneously it was time to take flight no matter what my neighbors were doing or what was promised in the efforts to restore the devastated building. All of my excuses for not moving and the weight

WHAT TO DO AFTER "I'M SORRY, IT'S CANCER."

of my procrastination were washed away. I had been there for too long.

For some reason, the flood, more so than the second cancer, was a major catalyst. Maybe it was just one too many nasty happenstances out of my control. I truly let go and let God (or the Universe, or the Matrix, or what have you). I let things unfold. I floated with the current, so to speak. And amazing things started to happen.

My inner voice told me that nature was what I needed and I took up kayaking. I spent a lot of time alone in Calgary's majestic backyard, the Rocky Mountains, and did something unprecedented and unexpected, surprising even myself, by kayaking alone from Invermere to Radium. I also took a trip to Whitefish, Montana and rented a cabin deep in the woods where I kayaked on the massive lake, solo. Maybe not so adventurous for the more outdoorsy of you, but exceedingly outside-the-box for an urban chicken like me.

I was displaced for three months, and stayed with various friends while living out of suitcases with my life's accessories in the trunk of my car and my belongings in storage. Apartments were at near zero vacancy rate and rents soared astronomically. I got to know my friends better and got an intimate glimpse into the lives of others after having lived alone for so long. I learned the meaning of living in the moment and tried to do so with grace and humor.

Somehow, money showed up from the strangest of places. I found a vastly upgraded little nest. Oddly enough, it is just what I had envisioned in my mind's eye over the prior few years; a balcony, a dishwasher (I haven't had one in over 16 years), a granite island to cook and entertain at, stainless steel appliances, washer and dryer in-suite, and the *pièce de résistance*—heated underground parking! I've never even had a covered parking spot in my whole life. It's micro-tiny, but adorable.

My brother once sent me a joke after yet another crisis. It is from the comical www.despair.com, a company that sells "demotivational" posters. On it was an image of a ship sinking with the caption:

MISTAKES
It could be that the purpose of your life is only to serve as warning to others.

We laughed. But I have often thought that if writing about my challenges or mistakes can serve as an early warning: STOP—DON'T BE

OBTUSE—LISTEN TO WHAT'S GOING ON IN YOUR LIFE, *before* a Titanic episode occurs in someone's life, then I've served the world in some small way.

This year was the most physically tiring of my life. But I am on a different trajectory. I am allowing more and controlling less.

Now, at the turn of a new year and a fresh start, take a peak at the worst best things in your life. And seize the day. Let the twisting tides take you down a new passageway—one that you've not previously permitted or imagined.

We have multiple realities at our fingertips. Which do you choose?

The Worst Best Things in Life
http://wp.me/p2ACw4-jG
lifebyheart.wandasthilaire.com

21

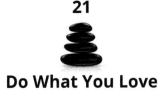

Do What You Love

Imaginary fences made of stone can be dissolved with the power of thought
'Shoulds' and 'musts' and 'have tos'
like dust
can be carried away in the winds of change

Shun boredom of the spirit

Build sand skyscrapers
Ride wild horses through canyons
Meditate with monks in Katmandu
Eat colossal sundaes for breakfast
Sing sonnets with gondoliers
Run with bulls in Pamplona
Fly to the west side of the moon
—Wanda St. Hilaire
Of Love, Life and Journeys

As odd as it sounds, cancer is the ultimate permission slip to fall in love with the mystery that life is. It is the consent form to do what you love *now*. This is your life we are talking about.

This is not a time to do the things you have always hated. Those things can wait—possibly forever. This is a time to be loving, kind, and extremely gentle with yourself. It is a time to play. A time to let go.

I have a cherished friend who was diagnosed with a chronic disease. In the name of healing, she chose to do everything that has been painful, extreme, and self-punishing with a strong theme of deprivation. I have pleaded with her to do the things she loves and only now after five years is this idea slowly sinking in as a possibility after tremendous suffering.

What have you given up in the name of duty and responsibility that you used to love to do? What lights you up? What are you passionate about?

What do you value most? What makes you happy? Focus on what brings you joy and makes your body sing. Write a list of at least ten things you value above all. How often do you engage in these activities or live the life you most cherish?

In Mary Oliver's poem, *Wild Geese*, she tells us: "*You only have to let the soft animal of your body love what it loves.*" The "soft animal" of your body knows what it wants; it knows what it loves and what it needs. We bend and twist ourselves like pretzels to fit the mold of society's norms, and of what our tribe expects of us, yet it may be completely contrary to what the soft animal—our heart—so desires. If we are performing a contortion act, cancer can bring us face-to-face with the fact that we are not doing what we love.

(*Wild Geese*[1]—An evocative cancer poem.)

Cancer reminds us that time is precious—especially now—so invest it in things that have meaning. By the time we find ourselves in a crisis of some sort, we may discover that we have given up a lot of the things we most adore. If we are out of touch with theses things the majority of the time, we need to make a lifestyle change and reevaluate our priorities.

It may not have appeared logical that I chose to go to Mexico, but when I made the decision to go to away pre-surgery and post-treatment, it was the best thing I could have done for my own sense of equilibrium, health, and happiness. I became a *human being* instead of a *human doing*.

In an excerpt of my letter to a friend:

> But I do know why this is the place of my soul. Aside from the ocean, the sun, the sand, the birds, the whales, the dolphins, it is the people ... do you know how many smiles I have received in one day? Nods? Holas? Today, a man carrying a large sack over his shoulder sang melodiously as he walked, yet he stopped his happy tune to say hello. How can one not feel better?

Stop wasting time. Do what makes you happy. Give yourself permission to do what you love. Grab life and wring every ounce of excitement out of it that you can. The clouds may be dark right now, but you can still dance in the rain.

---

1   http://rjgeib.com/thoughts/geese/geese.html

A powerful reminder
'Everybody Dies, But Not Everybody Lives' by Prince Ea
https://www.facebook.com/PrinceEa/videos/10154538480184769/

Article of interest about my post-cancer experience:
Vallarta: My Healing Place (Parts 1 and Parts 2)
http://www.wandasthilaire.com/pdf/PV%20Mirror%20-%20Healing%201.pdf
http://www.wandasthilaire.com/pdf/PV%20Mirror%20-%20Healing%202.pdf

The Feeding and Watering of a Soul
03/31/2015

"Ask her what she craved and she'd get a little frantic about things like books, the woods, music. Plants and the seasons. Also freedom."
—Charles Frazier

I was recently with Diane, a woman I had just met through friends, watching the sunset on the Bay of Banderas at my favorite spot on the beach. We were near the lava-like rocks and the Boy on a Seahorse statue and we chatted about life over our frosty to-go margaritas.

Diane asked me if I had ever been to Greece. Yes, twice to Athens and the Cyclades and the whitewashed islands are on my radar once again. She has been married for 25ish years and said she has always had a deep longing to see Greece, but her husband has no interest in it.

I got to thinking about what feeds the soul and I felt a bit sad that Diane (whom, as we uncovered in conversation, was my schoolmate for six years) has not yet experienced the unparalleled beauty and culture of Greece, even though the craving has been with her for three decades. Greece is likely something that would feed a part of her soul's need for that particular pleasure.

We are not taught to feed and water our soul as we would our gardens or houseplants. It is something we see as ephemeral and intangible, oftentimes ignoring it. Yet it is as important to our sustenance as any garden's harvest.

As children, we knew what fed our souls intrinsically. We would do it relentlessly, be it playing with Barbies, chasing frogs, reading Trixie Belden, or hitting a baseball. But then we were herded off into reality and the land of responsibility.

Feeding our soul equals pleasure. Possibly carried over from the Puritans and the centuries of religious influence, a lot of us believe pleasure equals guilt. But what if we are here to experience a whole lot more bliss than we allow ourselves? Why is Earth so incredibly bounteous if not to relish it with ridiculous amounts of joy?

Our soul whispers its desires to us, its requirements. If we do not listen, it may begin to niggle. If we continue to disregard it, our contentment wilts. When we starve it, our happiness withers.

If you seldom delve into what might nurture your soul, here are a few clues …

When you read something in a magazine or book that rouses you, pay attention to what catches your eye and makes you come alive. I am always drawn to magazine features with serene, minimalistic spaces of beauty, and images of foreign locales. Books with a philosophical angle awaken me and I love learning more about the mysteries of life and the human mind.

Music is like a colossal banana split for the soul. When I hear Latin music, I have a hard time sitting still. Walking into the corner bars on the streets of Old Havana, I could not have stayed seated if I tried. There is something about salsa and the *son cubano*[1] beat that brings my body alive and fills me with a sense of color.

Are there creatures or vistas that make your insides do flip-flops? I am always surprised when I ask someone if they would like to go whale watching and they reply with, "Nah, I've already seen them." There are never too many whale sightings for me. No matter how many times I've seen them, I always get excited each time I head out on the water to find them. I am ever gleeful when I see a dolphin, or turtle, or manta ray. Being on the ocean clears the cobwebs of nonsense from my mind in a way that nothing else can. What in nature makes you feel like a child seeing something for the first time? That is your soul's food.

When you overhear a conversation and you crane to eavesdrop (not in a gossipy way) what is it that makes your ears perk? When I hear conversations in Spanish or Italian, my heart leaps. I love the romance and the rolling singsong sounds of those languages. Something happens to me and it triggers an internal spark. One day I went out shopping with my friend Karen—a highly uncommon occurrence for me. Everywhere I turned people were speaking Spanish. She didn't notice, but I was acutely aware of it. It felt like the siren song of my yearning soul.

What subject makes your eyes dance and inspires you so deeply that you just cannot shut up? If you ask me about my trips to Italy—or almost anywhere—sit down and grab a drink. You'll be there a while. I love

---

1   http://en.wikipedia.org/wiki/Son_(music)

telling stories about the people I have met, the unforgettable meals I have eaten, and the amazing things I have seen.

What type of exercise comes naturally to you and makes you feel fantastic? I am not a Sporty Spice, so this one's not easy for me. But I discovered kayaking a few years ago and was surprised how I took to it like a duck paddling on a pond. The freedom of being on the water in a quiet, tranquil mode of transport that is so in touch with nature moves me. When I began Latin aerobics (vastly different from Zumba), I was hooked.

When you see a movie, what stirs and touches you? I remember watching *Under the Tuscan Sun* for the first time. It's not a poignant movie, yet tears trickled down my face for half of it. I knew it was because I saw myself in the main character. I adored Italy and had many moments of déjà vu there. I love *la dolce vita* and I could see myself living in that antiquated Tuscan casa, minus the scorpion. When Diane Lane had the fling with the dark, charming *Italiano*, she was me.

In the past few years I have had a thirst for learning. Recently it feels almost unquenchable and I think the reason is that my soul wants to sink its teeth into some serious study that will further my evolvement.

A client of mine told me last week that his wife says he suffers from PMS in the winter: Parked Motorcycle Syndrome. He is a big bear of a man and when I asked him what he felt when he rode his bike, his eyes glazed. He waxed poetic about the release, the smells along the highway, the fresh air, and the fabulous sense of freedom. Without a doubt, biking feeds this man's soul.

When we are obeying our soul's bidding, time becomes irrelevant. We are not concerned about the next task we have to do, or where we need to go. We savor the moment like a heavenly bite of hot, homemade bread slathered in butter.

A friend was a bit baffled about my recent trip—my 39th—to Mexico. How could I go when my current reality should not allow for a holiday? Should I not be a little more practical and hunker down? It *was* illogical. The thing is, my soul was quietly thirsting. It was salivating. It wanted to be amongst *mi gente*—my people. It needed Mexico for its survival, if only for a brief taste.

Interestingly, I was to experience a glaring paradox on this sojourn. I made the trip happen by booking the most humble stay of my travels.

During the trip I was invited, for the first time, to my friends' sprawling penthouse on the ocean with its 360-degree view and gorgeous contemporary comforts. At the end of the trip, I went to see the surreal, lavish castle of another friend's stay—a place I have walked by a hundred times, always wondering what lay behind the stone walls.

The juxtaposition was a bit jarring. I love luxury as much as anyone. But I learned something. Waking up in my small Mexi-room on the hard bed with its threadbare sheets, my happy heart was still grateful. I walked along the seaside silently sharing my gratitude list with the Universe each morning.

I was in the sweet frequency of my soul, and it was singing because I had satiated and honored it.

The Feeding and Watering of a Soul
http://wp.me/p2ACw4-ux
lifebyheart.wandasthilaire.com

22

Self-Talk

The thoughts of others are not you
But the thoughts you hold become who you are
Do not batter the child within
For she weeps with each blow

Dwell on your goodness
Bask in your courage
See the lush spectrum of the wildflowers you sow
over all you touch
—Wanda St. Hilaire
Of Love, Life and Journeys

I have been a student of psychology, spirituality, and self-help for many years, but since my second diagnosis seven years ago, I have been in intensive study. I have a burning desire to know why we get the results that we get in our lives. I have tried and tested an array of techniques and protocols and nothing has had the impact on my life more than changing my inner dialogue—my day-to-day self-talk. The most critical diet for health and happiness is what we feed ourselves in the content of our words—the conversations we have with ourselves.

I had tried affirmations many times before because every spiritual teacher states that our thoughts create our reality—and it never seemed to make a difference. But I dug a little deeper. The way I typically performed affirmations was to repeat them in the morning, and maybe again before bed. Without results, I decided affirmations didn't work, so I quit.

Then it dawned on me that if it took decades to create a bad habit, belief, or thought pattern, I wouldn't fix it with a couple of weak repetitions a day. The brain does not operate on a flip switch. I needed to make a concerted day-to-day effort to manage my self-talk and replace negative chatter with positive affirmations.

If this sounds like too much work, reconsider. You are going to dialogue with yourself all day anyway, so why not change it to a life affirming, happiness building *tête-à-tête*?

When we keep reiterating, in thought and in conversation, how sick we are, or how hopeless life seems, we will undeniably plunge our morale into a swamp. First and foremost when diagnosed with cancer, it is advantageous to sidestep a victim mentality.

Consider that your thoughts operate like a broadcast. The thoughts produce feelings and the feelings generate an energy you emote. If you find that hard to believe, think of how you feel when you are around an angry or bitter person. You palpably feel their swirling negative energy.

When you change your thoughts, you change your energy. I have discovered that positive self-talk increases my vitality and improves my mood significantly. People respond to me in a kinder manner when I am actively kind to myself.

With my self-talk campaign, I observed the words I said to people and the negative commentary running through my head on a daily basis. I then wrote out lists of upbeat affirmations. Because I get lazy about reciting them, I recorded them on my phone. I listen to them while getting ready in the morning and in the car when I am driving through the city between appointments.

Here is an example of simple daily self-talk to work with:

I love and accept myself
My body has the ability to heal itself
My cells are growing healthy and strong
I love and appreciate my body
I deserve perfect health
I forgive myself
I am unique and precious
I am valuable
I am energetic
I am triumphant
I am serene and calm
My immune system is healthy and powerful
I am important and I matter
While I sleep, I heal
I am grateful to be alive

I now nourish myself with love and joy
I will survive and thrive
I love and approve of myself
I lovingly forgive and release all of the past
I am healed and whole
I am enough

Self-talk is like a roadmap that sets the direction of your life. What you focus on expands. And what you repeat in your mind is, essentially, creating your truth.

Japanese researcher, Dr. Masaru Emoto, did groundbreaking work, which proved that water is deeply connected to human consciousness. Through a process of freezing water droplets, he discovered the crystals that formed varied greatly depending on the condition of the water.

When words or phrases like *gratitude, thank you,* and *I love you* were taped to the bottles of the water, the crystals were exquisite. Playing peaceful music, saying prayers over the water, and affixing lovely pictures on the bottles also had a positive impact on the beauty and shape of the crystals.

When phrases like *I hate you* or *I want to kill you* were taped to the bottles, the crystals were malformed and ugly. Water taken from polluted dams and waterways froze in the same way. And when heavy metal music was played to the water, the crystals showed discordance.

Consider with this mind-blowing concept, that our bodies are mainly water. Words of self-compassion and love heal. Words with negative resonance destroy.

Unfortunately, the masses (yours truly included) live too much of the time in the reptilian part of the brain where survival, fear, compulsion, and greed thrive. Dwelling here keeps us stuck. It blocks creativity and the connection to the inherent power within. It is where we spin our wheels in analysis, paralysis, and obsessive thinking.

Do not continually think and speak of illness and misery and what you do not want. Promise you will no longer be cruel to yourself in any way. Use your words instead for what you want: happiness, peace, health, and wellness. Self-talk your way to your healed, happy, and self-loving life, and remember—your cells are eavesdropping and responding in kind.

Water Crystal by Masaru Emoto/What the Bleep Do We Know?!
https://youtu.be/oQ5_9dzqNNs

Water, Consciousness & Intent: Dr. Masaru Emoto
https://youtu.be/tAvzsjcBtx8

The Taming of the Twerp
11/06/2014

"We have met the enemy and he is us."
—Pogo (Walt Kelly)

I found an old book published in 1982 called *The Inner Enemy: How to Fight Fair with Yourself* by Dr. George R. Bach. The header immediately caught my eye: 'Stop being ruled by that little twerp inside you!'

We've all got one—that twerpy inner voice nagging at us about one thing or another. Names for it vary:

The Inner Enemy
The Inner Critic
The Saboteur
The Enemy (meaning the devil in Christian corners)
The Dragon Within
Resistance
The Inner Bully
Ego
And plain, old-fashioned Guilt

Dr. Bach defines our Inner Enemy as the uncreative focus of our energies. *"It is our anger turned inward on ourselves."*

Sometimes it is much more than a nagging voice—it is a relentless roar with an unfathomable litany of abuse. We want acceptance from others, but we permit the pedantic Twerp to sing its songs of self-judgment. If anyone else ever said such things to us, we would likely terminate the relationship. But all too often we allow this part of ourselves to run amok and dictate far too much in our lives.

Few are immune. Les Brown is a world-renowned motivational speaker. I have been listening to his talks for some time and in one particular lecture he spoke about his experience with being told he had prostate cancer. Even as one of the most influential motivators, he was overcome by the voice of fear and skepticism just as strongly as any of us. He was bold enough to comically reveal some of the crazy things he did in abject terror for the sake of saving his life.

Wayne Dyer, for all of his self-help books and proselytizing on attitude, fell into a deep depression when his marriage failed and admitted to staying in bed once for three weeks.

Not even Jesus or Buddha were exempt.

There is always a consequence for allowing the nitpicking voice to rule unrestricted or for denying it altogether. It may be as seemingly benign as couch potato-ism or it could seductively lead us down the dark path to tragedy. On an almost weekly basis we see how the Inner Saboteur defeats countless actors, athletes, and musicians—people who appear to have it all. They seek to silence the voice with drugs, sex, and alcohol to the point of destruction and death.

The first line of defense is admitting that we have an inner voice that is not working for our best interests. We often dismiss the idea that we have an Inner Enemy. If it only creeps out in one area of our life, it is easier to ignore. We would like to believe we are Twerp-free and to present to the world as though we have our life together, but if we are honest with ourselves, we will most likely find evidence of its existence. The Twerp *loves* when we refute its presence or power because unacknowledged, it has carte blanche to freely maraud, harangue, and pillage our lives with glee.

Dr. Bach states in the book:

"Becoming aware of the Inner Dialogue, encouraging fair debate leading to decisions which reflect our own best interests, are crucial, *for the outcome of the Inner Dialogue determines the outcome of our life.* It makes the difference between success and failure, pleasure and pain, self-esteem and self-loathing."

It is *that* powerful. Once you succumb to the Twerp (believe its lies), it's a downward spiral.

How can the Dragon Within pull your life off course?

The most obvious tactic occurs when we try to make a significant change. Have you ever started a diet, taken up meditation, quit smoking, began an exercise routine, or tried to break a bad habit? The Twerp's backlash to a shift in the status quo can be torturous enough to stop even the strongest of us or send us running with our tail between our legs, back to the safety of the old parameters. Twerp abhors change.

Have you ever ...

- Called yourself a name or negatively labeled yourself?
- Habitually missed deadlines?
- Constantly lost things?
- Been prone to workaholism?
- Become a clumsy bumbler for no reason?
- Procrastinated in a big way?
- Berated yourself viciously?
- Let fear keep you from doing something fun?
- Overindulged on a regular basis?
- Had writer's or artist's block?
- Totally goofed off when you had something important to do?
- Talked yourself out of a really good idea?
- Felt irritated and angry for no apparent cause?
- Given up on love or a dream?
- Gotten sick right before an important event?
- Stayed at something or with someone you don't like or even despise?
- Doubted your ability to do something you know damn well you can do?
- Had perfectionist tendencies?
- Concerned yourself with the good opinion of others?
- Felt dread or anxiety when things are going too well?

If so, you're likely dealing with Twerp tampering.

Uncovering the voice is not always easy. The Twerp can be incredibly subtle and sneaky and prefers to keep a low profile. It hangs out in the subconscious and can leave you feeling mystified about unidentifiable angst.

Twerp keeps a running list of every rule our parents, teachers, culture, our church, and all authority figures have handed us. Conformity is its lexicon. It deftly catalogues every mistake, failure, label, criticism, embarrassment, heartbreak, betrayal, and shameful event. It is indefatigable in spinning the old stories 'round and 'round in our heads when the time to strike is ripe.

Do we come fully loaded with an Inner Twerp?

Without a doubt we are infected with viruses that begin shortly after our arrival on planet Earth. We are handed down half-baked belief systems and hear all types of messages that give the Twerp momentum. It starts at home; not necessarily out of malice, but of generational hand-me-downs and ignorance, and then proliferates with interactions from teachers, friends, and fellow students. Negative feedback, criticism, and bullying at school all feed the hungry Dragon. We download and store these messages in our operating system and Twerp guards them like Fort Knox.

The movie *What the Bleep do We Know?!*[1] brilliantly illustrates the significant damage the Twerp can do to us. Within the documentary is the story of a woman who has become embittered by a cheating husband, and how her Inner Critic negatively impacts her life and relationships.

Thankfully, we do have a supportive inner cheerleader that tells us "I can do it," "I am skillful," "I am intelligent." It is the motivator and inspiration behind our successes. It is our spirit and comes from the seat of the soul. It can warn us to stop doing something harmful, but if that voice attacks, it is definitely not coming from the higher self.

We war with the Twerp. We try to silence and smother it. We wrestle with it. We are disgusted by it. But I have begun to see that the voice is not the devil enemy we imagine it to be. It is the rejected, the hurt, and the scared part of us. Ironically, it is born in self-protection, yet set free to make tainted decisions and twisted declarations, it is capable of obstructing our best laid plans and can slowly and painfully fester into self-hatred.

Making peace with the Twerp is the best way to come to a détente. Years ago I worked with a therapist who suggested I name that nasty critic within. I called my Twerp 'Annabelle the Bitch'. Lately I have been negotiating with Annabelle (I dropped the bitch part—not the best way to build a friendship), and she's revealed some interesting, insider information.

I heard Elizabeth Gilbert, author of *Eat, Pray, Love*, speak about what she feels her biggest triumph is. She said it was the process of understanding the harsh voices within. She spoke to them and calmed them as she would her children. She told them to rest, to go to sleep, and that she would take care of them. She quieted them.

---

1   https://youtu.be/m7dhztBnpxg

What is your Inner Twerp trying to tell you? What poppycock is it selling you about you? Let it speak, and when it does: listen. Pay close attention to its stories rather than letting your monologues run unchecked, casting black clouds over your days. Call and counter its hogwash. Cry if need be. Rather than disown this influential part of yourself, discover what it wants and quell its fears. Befriend it instead of declaring a war that you won't win.

Ask the important question: is what that voice saying really *true*? Once we question and dismember the lies and warped perceptions of the Twerp, we can transform our relationship with it.

The Twerp is a formidable foe and the war within is the biggest battle we will ever face. The good news is that we have the power to call a truce. From a Jungian perspective, shedding light on our shadows dissolves the monsters we seek to keep hidden under the bed.

From all accounts, the payoff of acknowledging and reconciling with our demons is as unique and varied as snowflakes. When Liz Gilbert put hers to sleep after doing the work in an ashram, was it worth the effort? Well, let's see … after she left India, she found love in Bali, walked away from her journey with a worldwide blockbusting bestseller, and is a highly sought-after speaker with yet another bestseller.

While navigating life by heart, I have come to understand that the taming of the Twerp is the most crucial peace work we can ever achieve in life. Being gentle with ourselves; loving ourselves; having compassion for ourselves transmits like a satellite around us. It inspires and heals those within our reach. It can shift the outcomes in our lives: as within, so without.

Who knows what *your* payoff could be in an armistice with your Twerp? I propose you make an ally of your shadow. Whatever wonders await you, I wish with all of my heart that peace be with you, and with the wounded world at large.

The Taming of the Twerp
http://wp.me/p2ACw4-sX
lifebyheart.wandasthilaire.com

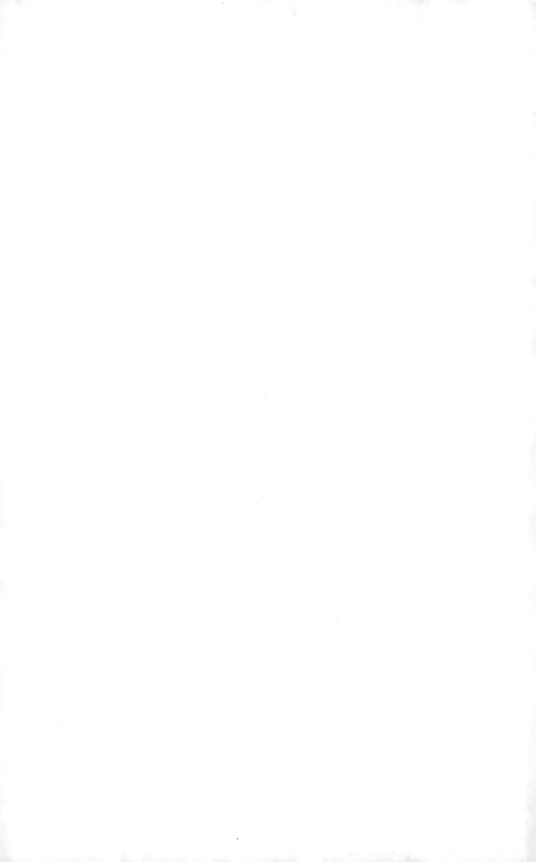

23

Attitude

"Having a great attitude and fierce faith in the face of cancer, at any stage, is not naiveté or denial. It is an excellent form of self-preservation and self-love."
—Wanda St. Hilaire

My friend Lynne was one of my cheerleaders upon my first diagnosis, then me with her, then her with me again. She was a head nurse at the hospital in my home city and had recommended her surgeon: the man who had performed her lumpectomy, and a trusted colleague she had worked with, side-by-side, for years. On the day we sat in the waiting room to first consult with him, I was gripped with fear, my nerves jangling in my ears.

The advice of others came to mind and I thought about the British-isms from my childhood.

"What in the hell is a stiff upper lip anyway?" I asked her.

We ended up in hysterics, contorting our faces in an attempt to form a stiff upper lip. The others in the waiting room looked at us as though they thought we were mad. It took everything I could muster to keep my anxiety under control and the laughter distracted my churning mind.

The first time I traversed cancer, I had an amazing attitude. As far as I was concerned, it was an anomaly, and I would come through with flying colors. The second time, I was angry—very angry, indeed. And utterly shaken.

I had been certain that after a twenty-year triumph, cancer had no more lessons for me. I had made adjustments in my life to ensure I would stay healthy and I had learned many things from the experience. A second diagnosis meant this thing was more than an anomaly. I was thrown into an epic existential crisis and it took time to pull myself together and adopt an attitude that would facilitate my healing. I could have suffered less by sooner accepting what was instead of being in resistance to the situation.

Having a good attitude does not mean bottling up emotions, being stoic, or faking it. It means believing in your healing, having faith, and keeping hope in the face of fear. When you are blue or angry, allow it. Who wouldn't be? But do what you can to stay optimistic. Find things to read or listen to that will inspire you and coax you out of a funk.

Give as little airtime to that which you are trying to escape and a lot of airplay to possibility and health. Behave as if you will completely heal. Don't deny; act as a well person rather than an ill person. Speak of plans for the future.

Attitude and beliefs go hand in hand. What is your perception of the world? What do you believe about illness and healing and more specifically—cancer? Beliefs are arbitrary ideas we consider to be true based on our upbringing, religion, cultural indoctrination, societal pressures, and trends. North American society believes in a seek-attack-destroy view of cancer whereby many other cultures use a gentler and less combative approach. Convictions are extremely powerful, but they can be transformed with awareness.

In *Anatomy of an Illness*, Norman Cousins said that because he did not accept his verdict, he did not get caught in the web of fear, panic, and depression that a serious diagnosis can spark. He did not deny the seriousness of the situation; rather he made it his objective to *defy* the verdict. He believed he had the power to change the outcome. He researched the biochemistry of emotions and their impact on health and experimented on himself.

My cousin, a farmer who spent long days in the fields, was diagnosed with stage IV malignant melanoma many years ago. He told me that he knew he had a choice to go down the dark road of despair or to hold an expectation of wellness. He decided life was pretty great and kept a positive outlook on the situation, veering away from gloom when it crept in. He is still here today to tell the tale.

Almost any doctor will tell you that your attitude is one of the biggest factors in your healing. Your will to live influences your physiology.

I had the rare opportunity to speak with a cancer pathologist recently. She told me that cancer cells, contrary to what we might assume, are actually rather beautiful. They have interesting geometric patterns, colors, and shapes. They are undifferentiated cells that have a mis-expression, which proliferates too far. She realized it might sound strange coming from a scientist who looks for disease all day, but she said she felt that instead of fighting cancer, we should bless it.

"When people are diagnosed with cancer, they need to come home to themselves," she stated. I was deeply moved by such a spiritual statement coming from a pragmatic scientist.

Instead of declaring war on cancer and creating a battle within, consider being for health and peace. Be a force for harmony and balance and come home to your precious self.

24

Gratitude

"Gratitude is wine for the soul. Go on, get drunk."
—Rumi

Gratitude? I was just diagnosed with cancer and it *sucks*. Agreed. It does suck. But one of the most compelling things you can do is give thanks ahead of an event—to say thank you for your healing, in advance, and feel it with your whole being.

Dr. Joe Dispenza has measured the physiological changes that gratitude creates in the body. A biochemical shift occurs which lowers the level of the stress hormone, cortisol, while the immune response goes up.

We are not hard-wired for an automatic gratitude response. We are largely conditioned to look for problems and to complain about the circumstances of our lives. But even in the face of cancer, there is always something to be grateful for each day.

If you are journaling through your experience, take a few minutes at night to review the day and say thank you for that kind nurse, the sunshine, the blue jay on the windowsill, or for your family's tender loving care. This practice reduces negativity. When you are thankful for what is good in your life, versus placing constant attention on the conditions and the fallout, it will boost your mood. You will be surprised at how many small things happen in one day to give thanks for. Track any positive happenstance. Observe the things you are learning and be grateful.

Say thank you frequently to those who are helping you, including the medical personnel. Bit by bit, as you exercise your "gratitude muscle," you will find yourself looking for the good. You will seek things to add to your gratitude list and as you assess your day with new eyes, you will have a sense of contentment, in spite of what you are going through.

It can be a tough concept to embrace when you are in the middle of a tempest, but blessing negative conditions is a powerful practice.

If you feel inclined, repeat these:

I bless this cancer for making me aware of changes I can implement for a better life.

I bless this cancer for the unexpected gifts it is bringing.

I bless this cancer for showing me the love I did not realize surrounds me.

I bless this cancer for bringing me closer to myself.

Remember to give thanks and appreciate your spectacular self for your strength, your courage, and what you give to others by sharing your journey with them.

TEDxSF | Gratitude
Louie Schwartzberg
https://youtu.be/gXDMoiEkyuQ

Gratitude and Tasty Turkeys
10/12/2014

"Piglet noticed that even though he had a very small heart, it could hold a rather large amount of gratitude."
—A.A. Milne
Winnie-the-Pooh

It's turkey time in Canada. I love this time of the year with its bountiful harvests of root vegetables and pumpkins and the deliciousness of a delectable turkey dinner. Thanksgiving Day can be traced back to 1578 and was declared a holiday in 1879 to celebrate the harvest and other blessings of the past year.

This weekend we are reminded to give thanks. But what about gratitude as a daily practice? I mean a conscientious everyday statement of blessings.

As I did laundry this morning, I remembered a young African athlete I met when I was 18 years old. I remember his name—Solomon Kondowi (I don't know if I've spelled it correctly). He was in Canada to compete in the Commonwealth Games and was being hosted by a friend's family.

What remained imprinted in my memory was his wonder and joy of what he saw in Canada. My roommate and I had him over for dinner one night and his face lit up in complete fascination as he described the washer and dryer he was able to use at his home stay.

"There are two big machines in their house. And you lift a lid, and you put your clothes in the machine. You shut it and push a button and it *washes the clothes for you*! Then you take the clothes and put them in another big machine right next to it and it *dries the clothes*! It's incredible!"

He was so thrilled with this experience and went on to describe how laundry was done back home by beating it on the rocks and washing it in the distant river. He also told us how he would be the star of his village with the new pair of Levi's the family had given him.

Most likely you have a washer and dryer at easy access in your home. This morning as I did laundry I got a small buzz of appreciation for those two "big machines." For 16 years, I had to go downstairs to a smoky, dingy basement to do my laundry with others. We shared one washer and one dryer in the building so laundry was *always* a production. Purposefully paying attention to all of the luxuries we take for granted and saying thank you for them reminds us that we likely have it pretty good, overall.

I know it may seem a bit trite and overstated, but there is a reason why most religions and spiritual practices promote thankfulness. As much as has been said or written about gratitude, there is actually nothing trite about it. It is a transformative force in human life.

Making gratitude a daily practice can shift your mood and bring in more optimism. I have started this once again to help change my attitude. This weekend I have set my phone alarm for every 15 minutes (while I'm alone). When it rings, I think of something or someone I am grateful for. It is an interesting exercise because it brings you back to the moment. Your focus is upon what is going on and what is good about right now.

When you actively remember to give thanks each day, you start becoming aware of the half-full glass. You complain less. It can nip envy and comparison in the bud.

Appreciation and gratitude can also have a calming effect over anxiety and worry. In stressful times, it is easy to forget the good. Jotting down the positives in a journal or sticking them on the mirror helps to break rumination on bad luck or hard times.

Remembering to thank others for anything they do for you improves relationships. Maybe you would like to write a note or call someone who has had a positive influence on you or how one small and seemingly insignificant act made a big difference to you at the time.

Noticing and appreciating the small beauties in nature takes our focus off of the material world. My spirits lift and my sense of wonder expands on my walks around the river. It keeps me mindful of the true values of my heart. My child-self sparks with awe when I see a woodpecker, warm sunbeams on the path, or a cloud that looks like a dolphin.

Cultivating gratitude can change circumstances. When we are grateful for what we receive and what we have, it allows life to give us more. It brings us into a state of grace.

I don't know *why*, but the Earth school is one of hard knocks. A very minute few of us escape unscathed. Right now, as I hang from a precarious ledge at mid-life, I need to remind myself that even though some challenges appear insurmountable, I am still very fortunate. I need not compare myself to the worst off, or the best off.

I admit to sometimes feeling defeated as a writer and wish for more readers (the raison d'être of all writers). But today, I say thanks to you for taking the time to read my blog. Thank you for your shares, comments, and uplifting responses. I thank you for making me feel like I am making a tiny difference.

Today I am grateful for …

You.
Sunshine.
Compliments.
Wellness.
Delicious food shared.
Being able to walk.
Loving friends.
Amazing family.
Love.
Breath.
Life.

And because tomorrow isn't promised, for today.

Gratitude and Tasty Turkeys
http://wp.me/p2ACw4-sk
lifebyheart.wandasthilaire.com

Down the Rabbit Hole

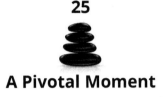

25

A Pivotal Moment

"Tell me, what is it you plan to do with your one wild and precious life?"
—Mary Oliver

Cancer presents an incredible opportunity—but you need the awareness to see it and the courage to grab it. Wayne Dyer called an occurrence like this a 'quantum moment.'

None of this is to diminish the fact that life happens. Things fall apart and come undone. Illness cannot always be prevented or circumvented and biology is a wild and fragile riddle. Sometimes we have no control of the ultimate outcome.

But if you return to "normal," to your old life, and continue to do everything the same way, you run the risk of getting the same results. Human beings are prone to complacency. For many of us it takes an unfortunate crisis or disaster to move us. Cancer is an especially painful two-by-four that clouts us out of our trances.

No matter the stage of diagnosis, you are being prompted to shift. You absolutely *do not have to*. However, you are being offered a space to make new choices, to create improved habits, to set clearer boundaries, to choose kinder thoughts, to build new beliefs, and to shift emotional states—if need be. You can decide to see your life through a different lens and take detours you never before dreamed. If you want an uncommon healing, you need to do some uncommon stretching out of your comfort zones.

What is cancer's personal message to you?

I guarantee, beyond a shadow of a doubt, there is one. If you look at cancer as a catalyst, it can be, in a peculiar way, inspiring. You can exploit it as a transformative reinvention of your life. As ironic as it sounds, if looked at with a subjective eye, cancer can be a savior—the ultimate course-corrector. As Dr. Joe Dispenza reiterates, we can actively and consciously create our lives, or we can live in reaction to it.

Bravely imagine fresh, spectacular scenes in your life beyond cancer.

Where are you living? What do you do in the mornings, afternoons, and evenings? Who are your friends? What or whom would you like to let go of in your life? Would you like to set out on a new adventure or enroll in a class? If you enjoy writing, pen scenarios you'd love to be in, fascinating conversations you may have, lists of dream tasks, places you will visit, and how you will feel through all those scenarios. Write about what you are looking forward to. Bring your future to life in animated color.

On my second cancer voyage, I refused to be pulled into a nightmare. Even though I did have surgery and treatments, and there were moments of abject terror along the way, I did the things I love most. Cancer presented an intense period of listening to my inner world, taking stock, and trusting, all in the midst of a cascade of advice, differing opinions, and a dicey financial outlook.

You can draw a line in the sand and choose not to let this experience be solely about the desolate landscape of hospitals, tests, pain, procedures, and appointments. I quite intentionally put the Charles Dickens quote in the beginning of this book as a beacon. This can be both the worst of times and the best of times.

Cancer is a teacher that leads us to a place of softness and vulnerability—sometimes on our knees. In Cancerville, you can let go of striving for a while. If you are open to embracing moments of quietude, it is the place of epiphanies. It is consenting to just *be*.

I travel solo and I have noticed that people will vacation with almost anyone just so that they are not alone. But I find that wandering in solitude is when some of the richest experiences occur. You unquestionably need support, but allow yourself time unaccompanied. Cancer has many things to tell you if you will set aside any concerns or discomfort you have with being alone with only your thoughts.

Now, you can discover your deepest truth. You will see the wonders of the world with new eyes if you so choose. Your reason for being here may become glaringly obvious. If you are still alive, you still have a purpose. In this pivotal moment, you can take previously untraveled paths. You can envision the authentic, one-of-a-kind you moving forward in a better, richer way, one specifically designed for your sense and sensibilities.

The Time of Your Life
08/21/2015

Open your eyes
wake from your dreams
and remind yourself that today
you will heighten your senses
to each kindness shown
to every smile
all things beautiful
vast or tiny
for none of these gifts are insignificant
in the eyes of the Universe
or the core of your soul
—Wanda St. Hilaire
Of Love, Life and Journeys

I spent a long, lazy, hot afternoon with my dad last weekend doing his favorite thing; philosophizing in a spiral deeply into the abyss—the nut doesn't fall far from the tree. We sat on a park bench and talked about illness. I said that I think the most effective thing a person can do when they are diagnosed with a condition is to do the things that bring them joy, firstly and foremost.

As my dad gets older, he is becoming acutely aware of what is most important in life. I know he feels time slipping away like sand in his hands. When he was still chock-full of testosterone and brimming with aggressive ambition—full of piss and vinegar, as they used to say—his perspective was a lot different.

One thing that ageing and crisis will do, if you are conscious and willing to listen, is get you to slow down and embrace enjoyment. We mostly live in a level of comfort that does not prompt big questions and reflection—until something monumental disrupts our complacency.

It would be absolutely impossible for you to know the impact and feel the deafening wallop of words like, "It's cancer," for a second time. Or "I'm sorry, she's gone," unless you've experienced them yourself.

One thing happens immediately; normalcy comes to an abrupt halt. The whirlwind of demands and "to dos" no longer have the same bearing on your life.

The year that I had a second diagnosis my life was a contradiction; it was a blend of agony and ecstasy. In the midst of confusion, I was able to step away from it and listen. And I heard joy calling my name. I *knew* in my heart of hearts that I had to do the things and go to the places that brought me the most happiness and delight if I was to heal. I didn't listen to the opinions of others or concern myself with what they thought of my decisions. I didn't let medicine dictate my life; I dictated how it could best serve me. It was not a time for hunkering into the world's ludicrousness. The lunacy could wait. It was a time for rest, and love, and laughter, and nature, and beauty, and kind healers.

But we don't need crisis or old age to slow down and savor life. We can do it right here, right now. If I could, I would let you see through the lenses of my rose-colored glasses, ones that have a filter crafted by the master teacher—adversity.

What I see is a gorgeous planet that wishes to be appreciated and honored, flowers that need to be ogled, and animals that are here to be observed with admiration.

I catch glimpses of dancing butterflies, iridescent dragonflies riding tandem, and busy bees dedicated to our wellbeing.

I watch imposing storms climax with full spectrum rainbows that summon awe and conjure pot-of-gold fantasies.

I see parks that ache to be played in, shape-shifting clouds that long to be watched, and trees that beckon us to sit under them with our blankets and pillows and books.

I hear rivers and streams gurgling and whispering their ionic therapy, if we only choose to sit near one in stillness.

I behold foreign places resplendent with history, rich with ethnic flavors and ancient mysteries that beg to be trekked and relished.

I see a cornucopia of whole food that wants to be sensually and slowly savored over lingering lunches with loving friends.

I notice strangers with whom we are meant to have synchronistic conversations and people who dearly need a random compliment, or an act of kindness, or one big radiant smile—one small gesture that could radically alter a bad day.

I listen to spontaneous offers to go for a walk in nature, or a drive to the majestic mountains, or to picnic on a hot summer's night; invitations that must not be refused because of a meaningless task that can wait.

I see homeless people who urgently need compassion and understanding, because there by the grace of God *go we*.

I sense embraces that want to be felt, love that wants to be expressed, and sex that yearns to be fulfilled, with white-hot presence and tingling pleasure.

I spot serious and solemn people who desperately need laughter and camaraderie to lighten them up and set them free.

I witness evidence of, and feel a benevolent and humorous intelligence that wants acknowledgment and gratitude, and invites us into a relationship so inconceivable that it will blow our minds.

And I spy with my little eye a burning passion inside of you that wants to be realized.

We tuck away our joy like our grandmothers saved their china for Christmas dinner. We don't allow ourselves the art of doing nothing but soaking up the beauty of life. But our bliss is meant to be lived now. *Today*.

What are your precious pleasures?

Like you, I squander fun and laughter for worry and survival and life's sometimes overwhelming "realities." Even though we all know we are leaving the Earth one day, we commonly act like we are superheroes who will live on to infinity in this form. We often think ... *tomorrow*.

What I would like for you to ponder today is the idea that we came here for unabashed joy. Not for seriousness, and guilt, and masochistic drudgery. Not for racing around in a frenzy that never ends and goes absolutely nowhere.

Pause.
Reflect.
Relax.
Listen.
Notice.
Smell.
Taste.
Savor.

Absorb.
Appreciate.
Breathe. Deeply and slowly. Right now.
Love life.

Allow yourself unbridled, uncommon, audacious glee. After all, what if that is why you chose to visit this weird and wild dot, suspended in space someplace in a galaxy called the Milky Way?

The Time of Your Life:
http://wp.me/p2ACw4-vK
lifebyheart.wandasthilaire.com

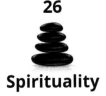

26

Spirituality

Does an angel wait nearby when you neglect her?
Or does she dissipate into the clouds to rest with other celestial creatures
until she hears you call?

This I would like to know when my heart is mute
For I want not for her to lose me in the murmurs of mortals
But to remain, in faith of my faith
—Wanda St. Hilaire
Of Love, Life, and Journeys

Spirituality could be considered your personal and unique relationship with creation. For some, cancer attacks the spirit. We may become angry and sullen because we feel we have been forsaken. I have friends and family who have concluded there is no higher power because something bad happened to them in the past. From experience, I would suggest that now is not the time to abandon your conversation with God or whomever you dialogue with. Dark times can bring us into a deeper relationship with the divine. Getting cancer does not make sense to our minds. But we have access to forces outside of ourselves if we seek them. Cancer can strengthen us and awaken our spirituality.

In 2010, I reevaluated my entire life from top to bottom. I went through a dastardly dark night and the bleakest moments were in the wee hours when no one else was around.

Faith is tested at a time like this and it may waver and wane. But even leaders, such as ministers and priests experience doubt. We can still live in the confusing mystery of our misfortunes while holding a mustard seed of faith.

When I need inspiration, I fill my mind by reading uplifting books and listening to motivational or spiritual teachings of leaders on YouTube. I feel buoyed and more optimistic afterward. Oprah invites a plethora of interesting authors and religious and spiritual teachers on her *Super Soul Sundays*. Ancient texts and the wisdom of the ages are available to keep you on hope's track.

Sometimes we try too hard. In her book, *Outrageous Openness*, Tosha Silver advocates the idea of inviting the divine into your life to guide you and to take the wheel, so to speak. Surrendering to the divine is a precious act in the cancer journey. Place your questions and worries into the hands of whomever you feel most connected to, be it Jesus, Buddha, the Virgin of Guadalupe, or Infinite Source.

It's vital you recognize that you are not waving a white flag and giving up, nor are you relinquishing responsibility. You are simply letting go and trusting a higher power to take the lead with a reprieve from worry. In surrender, you allow yourself to be freed from fear and you consent to being watched over and cared for by the unseen.

Ritual and prayer can assuage panic or mental paralysis. There is a loss of control in cancer; the rules you lived by may seem to disappear from underneath your feet. Some find comfort in creating a small altar with religious objects, candles, crystals, flowers, talismans, or *milagros*[1]. You may find solace in keeping a 'God Box' to place your prayers of petition and gratitude. You could choose a saint, archangel, deity, or animal totem to watch over you. Benedictine chants or classical music in the background can be soothing.

Your church may be a garden or a park. You can use affirmations, traditional prayers, angel cards, scriptures, a rosary, or beads for your prayer or meditation time.

We are taught to be goal-oriented and to strive and compete. Too often we spend our lives in survival mode rather than "thrival" mode. Dialoguing with the divine, in whatever form that may be for you, can bring comfort during this passage. Accepting direction from a higher power can strengthen you and bring a gentle whisper of grace into your life.

(For comfort and encouragement, you may want to listen to Joel Osteen on XM Sirius Radio or on TV on Sundays. His messages are always of empowerment and victory.)

---

1 *Milagros* is Spanish for miracles. Used here, they are tiny charms which represent things you are petitioning for.

27

Meditation and Mindfulness

"Meditation ultimately expands our sense of self and allows us to really enjoy each day ... to recognize that this human incarnation is fleeting and that the best way to move from this brief life to eternity is to take time to go beyond our boundaries and enjoy the vast cosmic dance."
—David Simon

The extraordinary benefits of meditation can no longer be disregarded. Even professional sports teams and the 'corporati's' CEOs are embracing the practice.

Excessive analysis makes the brain incoherent. Like many, I have a busy mind. I resist meditation because I am addicted to thinking and chewing on ideas and problems; however, I have learned that analysis typically solves little. An overactive mind can create even more confusion and worry, causing the mind to swirl around and around in an obsessive spin.

One of the biggest advantages of meditation for illness is the coherence factor. When we clear the mind and allow it to be still, it brings the rest of the body into unity, which is the optimal state for healing. Coherence means that when we give the mind a break from our incessant internal chatter it affords our body the chance to recalibrate.

Meditation is the best way to handle stress—with only positive side effects. It can shift us from a state of high anxiety to a peaceful, easy feeling without the need to medicate. It need not be a big production. Sitting on a park bench in silence is a meditation. Visiting the mountains and cloud watching is a form of meditation. You can begin with baby steps in small increments of time. Starting with five minutes is perfectly acceptable.

Mindfulness is simply a state of being aware of your surroundings and being in the moment rather than mulling over the past or fretting about the future. It is the power of now.

Meditation and mindfulness can significantly help with insomnia, fatigue, irritability, and digestive problems caused by nervous energy.

Another huge benefit for cancer patients is that it helps to diminish fear.

Meditating gives you access to the higher mind (the soul, the spirit, divinity). When you are in touch with your originating nature, you uncover the hidden. This is where infinite intelligence and wisdom reside. And it has a far grander and more exquisite plan than your physical mind can fathom. It can bring awareness and clarity and even epiphanies that elude us when we overthink. It takes us past the cacophony of worry to the sweetness of peace of mind.

To Be or Not To Be
10/04/2012

This time that I have been granted
to listen to my heart
tells me all its secrets ...
reveals its desires in shadowed curves
opens the doors of my imagination
germinates seeds of generosity
and heightens my senses to the surrounding beauty

Stop ...

Listen

And these gifts shall too be yours.
—Wanda St. Hilaire
Of Love, Life and Journeys

When was the last time you allowed yourself space—serious space—for just *being*? For pure quietude?

Western society has very little use for being. Doing is the measure of one's worth. I know I'm not the only one who struggles with "being time" in Calgary, the city of money and action.

When I've been told that I need to meditate, I think, *cripes*. Now I've got to sit in a lotus position (which my dry, twig-like body hates) and do some convoluted breathing exercise, while trying not to notice that my legs are going numb.

But fortunately I've discovered that my best meditating comes in the grandeur and bounty of nature. Lately I've had a constant craving for time outdoors in nature and nothingness and the weather has been perfect for it. Last weekend I spent both afternoons in a slow stroll and then sat on a riverside park bench.

Watching fall leaves floating freely down the

river and dancing in the wind ...
Observing ducks bobbing underwater for food ...
Listening to noisy magpies arguing ...
Stretching out with the warm Indian summer sun on my face ...
Embracing stillness.

In 16 years, I'd never seen a fish jump in the shallow Elbow River near my home and thought that it would be a treat to see one. I drifted off and when I awakened, the bugs were buzzing above the river. Lo and behold! A large fish leapt out of the water in front of me.

It was suggested to me as "homework" that I spend a few evenings under the stars to just sit and observe. I don't have a backyard or even a balcony, so the night before the full moon, I grabbed a pillow and found a bench facing the bright light of the moon in my neighborhood.

Firstly, it was impossible to see the stars with so much light in this downtown location. Secondly, I didn't realize how much traffic actually whizzes past my corner at 11:30 p.m. And thirdly, passersby were like curious cats and wanted to know what I was doing. So much for quietly bonding with the galaxy!

I wasn't prepared to give up on the idea. The next evening I decided to head out of Dodge. I went down the Bragg Creek highway and found a deserted side road. As I meandered, three deer gracefully made their way across the roadway in front of my car. I found a vacant little cul-de-sac, ideal for my foray. Then I became too scared to sit alone in the darkness and silence.

I backtracked to a park in Discovery Ridge where the stars and now full moon were perfectly visible and I set up the deluxe folding chair I carry around with me everywhere.

I was bundled up in my Lundstrom winter parka, cozy and warm, but antsy. I stared at the moon. I tried to figure out which constellation was what. I wriggled. I rearranged.

And then, there it was. A spectacular display of the mesmerizing aurora borealis. It spread and undulated across the heavens for at least 20 minutes. I was first awestruck and then deeply moved. I felt it had shown up just for me.

During my first long-term winter writing stint in Mexico 13 years ago, I lived off the beaten path in a rustic little house that I called Casa

Rosita. The walls inside and out were a soft-washed pink and in the middle of the house was a small courtyard with flowers and a chirping gecko where I hung a hammock and ate my meals al fresco.

I had no phone, no Internet, and no TV. At first, my chattering mind went into overdrive in the drubbing silence. But after a time, I embraced the hush and my mind blissfully paused. I spent many evenings in the hammock watching the one palm tree above me sway while the moon made its journey across the night sky. The peace of *being* was a most precious period of rest from the crazy-assed world.

What's interesting and oh-so wonderful is that as you relax, you attract. One's face and body unclench and hard edges and lines soften. The protective wall dissolves and vulnerability shines through, letting in smiles, compliments, and goodness. Rigidity becomes more fluid; the harsh boundaries of how things must be or should look begin to blur.

I mentioned my nature craving to my acupuncturist, Obi. She said maybe the time has come to just *be* for a while. Needles sticking about everywhere, she exited and left me with time for contemplation.

I have been a doer my whole life. I have been on one mission or another for as long as I can remember. My brain wants to create, develop, fix, and arrange. But in a whirlwind of doing, it is hard to assess where we stand. If we live life by rote or get caught in a habit of busyness, how can we know if we're on track or off the rails?

Knowing the tremendous benefits from my time at Casa Rosita, a period of reflection and *being* after a frenzy of doing is massively appealing, yet sounds all but impossible in the face of my current reality. When I considered allowing a window for some downtime, it brought out a nasty and relentless voice—chastising, warning, goading, threatening. The minute I reached for a respite—a little breath of the divine—the voice of the diabolical sought to destroy it.

In *The Art of Doing Nothing*[1], Véronique Vienne extols the virtues of the art of waiting. When we find ourselves at a lull in the pursuit of tomorrow, rather than grab the opportunity to take a breather, we feel impatient and frustrated. She says one of our worst fears is to be left behind as the world rushes toward its destiny.

I don't necessarily want to pull an Eckhart Tolle[2] by sitting on a park

1 http://www.randomhouse.com/book/183869/
the-art-of-doing-nothing-by-veronique-vienne-and-erica-lennard
2 http://en.wikipedia.org/wiki/Eckhart_Tolle

bench for two years, but a gap of time to just allow life to be what it will be sounds gloriously restorative.

In the midst of chaos, is *being* the answer? I can't afford the time to just be, you may think. But then again, maybe you can't afford *not* to invest the time to stop a wee while and discover a speck of magic in the power of stillness.

To Be or Not to Be
http://wp.me/p2ACw4-ab
lifebyheart.wandasthilaire.com

28

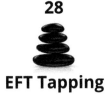

EFT Tapping

"Just like there's always time for pain, there's always time for healing."
—Jennifer Brown

Emotional Freedom Technique is a weird and wonderful meridian tapping method that I learned when I went to live in Mexico the winter after my treatments. Maraya, the gorgeous (inside and out) American girl I had rented my casa from, saw I was struggling emotionally. She had learned EFT and had seen amazing results in her life by diligently using this practice.

It seemed like such a bizarre technique that I didn't take the concept seriously at first. I found it hard to believe that something so simple (and odd) could help with both physical and emotional pain. As I learned more and read how it was being used for Post Traumatic Stress Disorder, with excellent outcomes, I began to practice it.

There is a lot of research and science behind EFT and many experts in health and self-healing endorse it. The technique was developed by Gary Craig and is a combination of psychology blended with lightly tapping acupressure points on the body to release trauma—a type of energy psychology. It can help reduce pain, diminish fear, eliminate phobias, clear limiting beliefs, aid with weight loss, and greatly lower your stress response.

EFT facilitates healing by stimulating and clearing blocks in the body's chi or energy meridians and the effects can be long lasting. This practice is so effective it has been used for trauma after mass shootings and in Rwanda post-genocide. It is being used on soldiers suffering with PSTD after their return from duty with results that traditional psychology and psychiatry is not achieving. It alleviates the pain of difficult or traumatic memories; even memories that we may not know are affecting us.

I have followed Nick and Jessica Ortner since they began their EFT Tapping Summits and have watched their documentary film, *The Tapping*

Solution. Nick has also written a book of the same name. Their organization has done much to spread the word about the healing benefits of EFT worldwide.

I discovered Brad Yates on YouTube, and I follow along with his various videos. He frequently uploads new content related to all types of issues and his style is comforting and warm.

What I have experienced with tapping is that it brings me back down to an even keel if I find myself flying high on anxiety. Equally, when I am feeling low, it brings me back up to equipoise. What's incredible is that EFT works as well or better than pharmaceuticals. It is easy to do and has no negative side effects. You can do it on your own at any time, following along on YouTube videos from a wide selection of practitioners.

A big part of physical pain is emotional in its roots. For instance, with my own diagnosis, I had strong emotions around being a single woman going through the cancer experience for a second time alone. I was disappointed and angry at myself, the system, and God. Tapping helped.

Set aside skepticism and give it a try. Using effective techniques like EFT tapping enables you to use your own innate ability to heal. It is free, easy, and can be done anywhere.

Tap your way to health and serenity.

The Tapping Solution YouTube channel: https://tinyurl.com/legmy32
Nick and Jessica's website: http://www.thetappingsolution.com

Brad Yates YouTube channel: https://tinyurl.com/lx6gtat
Also, you can visit his website at: http://www.tapwithbrad.com

If you would like to try tapping with a spiritual aspect to it, visit Robin Duncan's YouTube channel at: https://tinyurl.com/me35ktz

In case you are unable to search for what you need, I have created an EFT Healing Playlist for you here: http://tinyurl.com/zcjspv6

29

Visualization

One must not forget that recovery is brought about not by the physician,
but by the sick man himself. He heals himself, by his own power,
exactly as he walks by means of his own power, or eats, or thinks,
breathes or sleeps.
—Georg Groddeck
The Book of the It, 1923

Many years ago I learned about visualization in a book by Shakti Gawain called *Creative Visualization.* Professional athletes, musicians, actors, surgeons, and business leaders use this technique worldwide. Olympians use it to envision their winning performances. It is the art of visualizing or mentally imagining your future intentions in full living color, or as Dr. Joe Dispenza prefers to call it, rehearsing.

Scientific studies have proven that the subconscious mind does not decipher between what is imagined and what has really happened. This is what makes visualization such a powerful technique, if it is done with consistency. People who only *visualize* practicing the piano become better at playing and people who visualize performing a sport actually become physically stronger.

In essence, visualization is a way to "trick" the mind into believing the experience is happening. If you have trouble believing that the mind can affect the body's chemistry and physiology, all you need to do is think about self-pleasuring. It all begins with a scenario conjured up in the mind that your body believes is real because of your vivid fantasies. Your body quickly responds. So too with active, focused rehearsal and visualization of perfect health and all that you will do in that state of being.

Visualizing or rehearsing your recovery and health is an effective way to empower yourself in the journey and you only need to spend 5 to 10 minutes a day to do it effectively. It is best to be in a quiet place with no phones, computers, or televisions. If you need to, hang a *Do Not Disturb* sign.

Some cancer patients prefer images of creatures eating the cancer and others of assassins killing or blowing up the tumors and cells. I am not big on violence, so both times I envisioned fairies entering my bloodstream and, like picking berries, plucking out anything that looked suspicious. I imagined them carrying off any errant cells in small buckets out into space—I prefer pretty, gentle things. In *Creative Visualization* the 'Pink Bubble' technique is outlined. In it, you picture placing the cancer cells in a pink bubble that floats off and disappears into the ether.

After that, imagine yourself in perfect health. Speak to your body with compassion. Your cells hold consciousness and will respond. See yourself doing the things you love—be it mountain climbing or tango dancing. How will you feel? What events will you attend? Will you run a marathon or kayak on the ocean with dolphins? Will you travel to Katmandu?

Create a movie in your mind where you watch yourself play the starring role. Use smell, sight, sounds, tastes, feelings, and sensations when you rehearse and imagine. See yourself happy, robustly healthy, and energetic.

Practice positive emotions. Your body does not know the difference between a real emotion and one you are fabricating during your visualizations of wellness. As Dr. Joe advises us in his books, you do not wait for the healing to feel your wholeness and wellness; you feel it ahead of the event.

In the fall of 2002 I was on a writing sabbatical and not earning a wage. I began to fantasize about winter in my beloved Mexico, but by all appearances, I would not be going anywhere, except perhaps a local wave pool. One day I stumbled upon a book at the library called *How to Make the Impossible Possible* and I took it home. It was a reminder about the power of visualization, something I had used successfully in the past.

And so, I began a daily practice of a short visualization. I saw myself sitting at my favorite seaside coffee shop, Mundo de Café. I sipped the dark Chiapas espresso. I smelled the salty sea air. I savored chicken tacos smothered in salsa *verde* and lime-drenched guacamole. I felt the warm sun on my skin and imagined it becoming golden. I heard the birds squawking and listened to the high waves crashing on the shoreline. I felt the wind on my face and the spray of the water on my legs as I sat on the bow of a boat. I watched whales breach and dolphins play and pelicans dive. I let the excitement and joy of being in my happy place bubble up.

Within six weeks of beginning the visualizations, in the most bizarre and unexpected of circumstances, I had a ticket to Mexico for an all-expense paid two-week vacation. It was pure magic.

Visualize from a space of gratitude. Do not think about the hows. Take the time to create and imprint a positive outcome in your mind. I implore you to make this a fun part of your day. Do it with optimism for what will be, rather than from desperation or disappointment. If this feels like a chore, don't do it. However, if this resonates, practice with commitment. It is only effective when done repeatedly and regularly.

A great time to do affirmations is after visualization while you are in a relaxed and confident state. Simple declarations of "I am" such as, "I am healed" are effective.

Louise Hay says, the most powerful affirmation for all problems is, "I love and approve of myself." Leave affirmative notes on mirrors, the car dashboard, or fridge for a potent visual reminder of your wellness.

There are a myriad of guided healing visualizations on YouTube. I love the uplifting 'Manifest Three Wishes' visualization below and use it frequently. In it, you imagine three things you want to see come true. It is a soothing 10-minutes away from the world. (I use 3 stones I picked off the beach. You will see what I mean after you listen to it.)

Manifest Three Wishes Meditation
https://tinyurl.com/lddqg9d

If you would like an explanation of the power of setting intentions through visualization, Dr. Joe Dispenza explains it perfectly here: Defining Intention (27 minutes) https://tinyurl.com/kw9dx7u

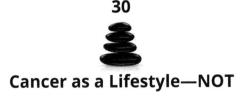

30

Cancer as a Lifestyle—NOT

"Stop taking identity in illness and start taking identity in wellness."
—Nina Leavins

Do yourself a huge favor. Don't join Club Cancer.

I was at an appointment with a doctor at a privately funded breast cancer clinic and she asked me if I was interested in a new group that was being formed for women with a triple negative diagnosis. Apparently a small circle of women were disappointed that a special group had not yet been created for the 'Triple Negatives' and they felt left out. (This means that the tumor tested negative in the pathology report for estrogen, progesterone, and HER2 receptivity.)

"What? Why would we need a special support group?" I said.

She suppressed an eye roll as she mumbled, "I don't really know."

When you hunker down into cancer victim mentality, and digest every little bit of bad press about your type of cancer, wearing it like a badge of honor, you are headed down a slippery slope. As long as you are alive, you are a survivor. Create a positive statement about your cancer journey; there is at least one good thing that cancer has inspired you to do.

Don't become too attached to the attention and care you are getting because of what you are going through. It is a wonderful thing while you need it, but if you become too dependent on it, your healing can be impeded by the emotional payoff.

My cousin's husband is a chiropractor with a deep interest in the mind-body connection. I asked him to tell me the best healing story he's heard so far from his patients. He said a man had come in with a note on his chart about a history of colon cancer and he inquired on its status. His patient was a no-nonsense type and replied that it was gone.

"What did you do to heal?"

The man said he had been given the diagnosis and recommendations for treatment. He was not impressed. He was sent to a support group as well. He said that he attended a meeting, listened to the whining and sad tales and walked out. He said he decided then and there: *This is nonsense. I am not doing this. I do not have this disease!* It may sound absurd, but part of the healing process is a firm, non-negotiable decision to be well. He was later declared cancer-free, minus treatment.

You can spend your life going from medical test to medical test for each ache, ever seeking that rat bastard, cancer. And it will drag your morale into the gutter. "Chronic" cancer must be monitored, but try not glom onto *my* cancer, *my* oncologist, *my* treatments, or *my* drug regime as though it is your new identity. You are you, not cancer. It is only the new you if you reinvent your life that way. Negatively programming your mind to revolve around illness and being hyper vigilant and in constant terror of cancer can affect your body, your peace of mind, and your spirit.

We have watched women exhausted and worn down from treatment with blisters on their feet in races and runs for the cure. Before you burn yourself out on a crusade and jump on the cancer bandwagon, research the organizations you are rallying for.

What I discovered in my research on breast cancer and cancer organizations is:

- In the breast cancer 'Pink Ribbon' world, there are *zero* allotments in their multi-million/billion dollar campaigns to support breast cancer patients who legitimately require financial aid.

- The percentage of funds that are directed to research and go to high salaries and operating costs are public knowledge, if you dig. Most of the organizations I researched were at over 50% in administration and salary allotment. Personally, I would rather support small local foundations with hands-on programs and funding with grants for cancer patients rather than rally for emblematic greed-based operations.

- As previously mentioned, research on acupuncture, homeopathy, naturopathy, nutrition, natural supplementation, and complementary medicine is not funded.

- These organizations will not support a scientist who has discovered a non-patentable cure. If there is a conceivable cure for your cancer, are you sure you want to support an organization that is uninterested and unwilling to invest in valuable research that could potentially save your life?

Before you deplete your body in a race or drain your funds, be sure you understand what you are supporting in the Club Cancer World.

Cancer is an unwanted guest that disrupts the harmony of all in its wake. Do not let it take up permanent residence in your life. Choose your words wisely, for they become your reality.

I am not cancer.
I am not my illness.
I am a strong survivor.

31

Random Acts of Kindness

"Be the miracle you seek."
—God
Bruce Almighty

When author Cami Walker was trapped in a mess of misery over a diagnosis of multiple sclerosis, she was given an unusual "prescription" from an African friend. Give away 29 gifts—something as simple as a compliment—in 29 days. The premise is that when you focus on what you have to give rather than your own despair and lack, you open up a space for abundance and healing. She documented her experience in a book of personal essays.

Even though you have been given a diagnosis and your life has been turned upside down, you still have a lot to give. I do not mean taking on the care of others. I'm suggesting small gestures that will uplift you. It could be a note of encouragement for someone you sit next to in a waiting room. It may be a cup of tea you buy for someone in a café. You might purchase a $1 lottery ticket and leave it with a note at a convenience store.

It is normal to become self-focused in the midst of cancer and I have reiterated the importance of self-care, but when we shift our attention off of our own tribulations to an intention of performing random acts of kindness it can help take the emphasis off of cancer. When you give, you are closest to the divine aspects of yourself. Again, if it feels like a hassle—don't do it. But if the mood strikes, try it on for size.

Jim Carey says: "The effect you have on others is the most valuable currency there is." I try to live this every day as my truth.

Free e-card service for random acts
http://www.wandasthilaire.com/ecards.php

Premeditated Acts of Kindness and Purpose Driven Beauty
03/30/2013

Nothing else counts in this life
if our heart knows not the song of love
generously scattered over all we touch
—Wanda St. Hilaire
Of Love, Life and Journeys

Who didn't love the movie *Pay it Forward*? (Okay, aside from the really sad part). We are moved when we witness people step out of self-absorption and pay attention to the plight of others to commit acts of kindness. When a moment of random compassion ripples through the pond of humanity great distances, it is even more awe-inspiring.

On a break during a Calgary Philharmonic Orchestra[1] presentation of Beethoven and Brahms, my friend Pat and I discussed the kindness of others. We were sitting in a semi-private balcony, compliments of my acupuncturist and her partner. It was a poignant performance featuring knighted pianist, Sir Joaquín Achúcarro, who astounded us with his one-handed recital of Brahms.

We were grateful for the gift of the music—and the privacy, because I kept disrobing due to hot flashes—and I pondered that maybe December 21, 2012, rather than heralding the end of the world, was the beginning of a new era of compassion.

Personally, in the past year, I have been the recipient of many acts of over-and-above kindnesses. My Momentum (school) mentor passed along my websites and writing to *her* mentor shortly after we began working together to garner his opinion. A business coach and writer himself, he loved my writing and made an offer to mentor me for as long as I wanted. He has become my biggest fan and tirelessly sends me inspiration, advice, and positive feedback—all out of the goodness of his heart.

I have received numerous services, both business and personal, on a website called Fiverr whereby many of the providers have not only given

---

1 http://www.cpo-live.com/main/

a lot for the $5 they get, but they have gone well beyond the confines of the gig to give more of themselves as an act of service.

My wonder boy proofreader and designer, Ryan, whose honesty is astonishing, refuses to charge me if the work I send is under 10 minutes, and my hair stylist gives me a pro-rated fee for her services that I did not ask for, but immensely appreciate.

The other day while writing at a café, I noticed a stunning girl of about 30 texting and reading. Before she left, she came up to me to tell me that she had been watching *me* and had debated about coming over, in case I thought she was a freak, but that she really wanted to tell me she thought I was beautiful. Feeling especially low that day, I told her she had made an excellent decision and that I much appreciated the compliment. It made my day and lifted my flagging spirits.

Pat said she had observed a mother and child in a store earlier in the week. The little girl was admiring a Barbie and was notably well-mannered. Another woman had also been watching them and asked if she might be able to buy the little girl a Barbie and her mother agreed to it. The benevolence of the gesture moved Pat.

That week Pat had also been the recipient of a random act from a stranger and was touched and surprised. When someone grants us their kindness in a moment we most need it, we feel seen. We feel like we matter.

I first began actively planning random acts after an exercise we were asked to do in a development course at Personal Best, which was facilitated, and gifted, by my friend Lynn. I had so much fun that I went on a rampage, anonymously buying coffee for strangers, leaving money on park benches with notes, topping up expired meters, and so on. One man was insistent on knowing who had bought his coffee and invited me to his table to ask why I had done it. It inspired him to make a plan to do the same.

But as is human nature, my random acts became rather, well, random. In 2011, I learned of a 29-Day Giving Challenge[1], joined it, and blogged about it. It was founded by Cami Walker who wrote a book[2] about a "prescription" she had been given by a medicine woman to change her focus on her health challenges to a focus of giving.

---

1   http://www.29gifts.org/
2   http://www.29giftsbook.com/

The selfish upside of random acts of kindness is the boomerang effect or the karmic benefits. Last month on what I now call Lucky Corner, I had said no to a homeless man who had asked for money. I had $20 left for the balance of the week and needed it. But halfway down the block I heard a voice say, *give him some money*. Really? Geez! I don't have much. *Yes. And not just change.* I turned around and much to his surprise, gave him half of what I had.

Two weeks later, I walked out of the same store, once again, with not much in my wallet or bank account. I saw a small white envelope on the ground and heard that same voice say, *pick it up*. I obeyed. As soon as I did, I knew there was something for me inside. And there was. $60 cash. Last week I won $50 there, and then another $10 on my lotto tickets, hence, Lucky Corner.

The other selfish part of giving is how good it feels. According to the Random Acts of Kindness Foundation[1], scientific studies have shown that we release serotonin, the neurotransmitter that elevates mood, when we perform an act of kindness and that it boosts our own immune systems. It is why volunteering and mentorship are so popular. If we are giving out of a heart-driven sense of generosity, the pleasure we generate gives us a feeling of wellbeing.

When we adjust our focus off of our own miseries to serving others, it pulls us away from the quandary we are in. And no act of kindness is too small. We have absolutely no idea how one small act, one compliment, one helping hand will affect another human being.

Stories abound of situations where one brief word of encouragement or gesture of compassion prevented a suicide. Of utmost importance is the fragility of teenagers who may be in a black pit of despair and need kind words or someone to listen and understand without judgment. Here is one poignant story from a hair stylist: *It Only Takes A Moment*[2]

It only takes a moment to make someone's day. Sometimes when the people closest to us do not see our pain, a stranger's goodness can make a massive difference. The next time you feel an inner nudge to compliment someone or do something nice, don't doubt yourself. Just do it. Your nervousness or reticence will be eradicated by the response.

I firmly believe that the reason unconditional kindness and compas-

---

1 http://www.randomactsofkindness.org/
2 http://daymakermovement.com/about/our-story/

sion feels so good is because it is one of the fundamental fuels of love, and that love, no matter how trite it sounds, is *the* answer.

55 Ideas for Premeditated Acts of Kindness

- Give a stressed out stranger a small bouquet of flowers.
- Help an elderly person with something: crossing a street, carrying groceries, etc.
- Leave $2 at the lotto-checking machine with a note: A random act of kindness for your winning ticket.
- Leave money in laundry machines.
- Buy something you really, really want (can be very small) then give it to someone else.
- Hold the door or elevator for someone who is at a distance from the door.
- Clean snow off of someone's car.
- Leave money in a library book.
- Make it a habit to pay attention to those around you who may need assistance.
- Make someone a CD of moving love songs.
- Bring a single or elderly neighbor dinner one evening.
- Tell someone they have inspired you or that you admire them.
- Promote someone you believe in with their efforts at their small business.
- Write out your best recipe and give it to someone who would appreciate it.
- Tape a sign in a public bathroom – *You are gorgeous. Yes! I mean YOU.*
- Pay for a coffee/latte and tell the barista to give it to whomever orders one next with the message that it was a random act of kindness.
- Buy someone's train or bus ticket.
- Buy your boss flowers and say thank you or tell them you think they are a creative genius or an amazing mentor.
- Say something nice to an overworked clerk in a store.
- Set up a lemonade stand in a park on a hot day and give away lemonade and hugs (how good will *you* feel afterward?).
- Give away a computer or cell phone you no longer need.

- Offer to make a colleague lunch the following day.
- Pay for the order behind you at a fast food drive-thru.
- Make someone a fabulous YouTube playlist: great music, inspiring stories, funny videos, cute animals—whatever will make them smile.
- Give someone a little box of Timbits (if you're a Canadian!).
- Tell a child or teenager something absolutely wonderful about them (they will never forget it).
- Sing to a small child.
- Send a card to someone struggling with an illness or disease to tell them you think they are courageous and strong.
- If you are a woman, smile and say something nice to an elderly man. If you are a man, smile and say something nice to an elderly woman—ageism is too prevalent in this society.
- Smile at everyone you pass by for one whole day.
- Send a teenager a card telling them who they are makes a difference to the world.
- Hug someone who has given you amazing service.
- Take a friend and go to a chemo ward or radiation ward and deliver a (real) chocolate and a smile or hug for everyone.
- Send your mum or dad a letter of all the reasons why you love and appreciate them.
- Write a love note of appreciation to your spouse and leave it in a surprise location.
- Give a chocolate bar to a taxi or bus driver.
- Leave money on a park bench with a note to cheer someone up.
- Post a letter of appreciation to a police station or fire station.
- Leave a car wash ticket in an envelope with a note on someone's dirty car.
- Drop by a seniors' home with roses or balloons and give one to each resident.
- The next time a homeless person asks you for money, give what you can with a big smile and "have a wonderful day."
- The next time you see a homeless person pushing a cart, stop and give them a $5 coffee card from the local coffee shop.
- Bring a box of donuts into a police station.
- In colder climes, give socks out to the homeless around a shelter.
- Compliment a stranger.

- Buy a case of cold water on a hot day and give out bottles to homeless where they gather.
- Give a stranger a movie pass.
- Leave a small potted flower on a neighbor's doorstep.
- Buy a roadside flag person/worker an ice cream cone on a hot day.
- Bring someone at work who needs appreciation some flowers.
- Call someone you haven't talked to in a while to tell them you love them.
- Leave the coin in a shopping cart for someone to find.
- Tape money to a vending machine with a note – Free treat on me!
- Take your good "one day" clothes to Value Village/Goodwill.
- Post a card or handwritten letter to a friend or family member in the mail.

Entertain the idea of random acts of kindness as a way of life. You will be the change you wish to see in the world!

You Get What You Give
https://youtu.be/k16sC7_H30E

Premeditated Acts of Kindness and Purpose Driven Beauty
http://wp.me/p2ACw4-eS
lifebyheart.wandasthilaire.com

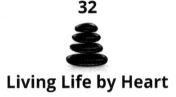

32

Living Life by Heart

To live is the rarest thing in the world. Most people exist, that is all."
—Oscar Wilde

Do you want to live? That's a strange question to ask since you are reading this book, but some people—in the privacy of their own pain-filled psyches—do not. They pretend for the sake of their loved ones, but they have resigned to cancer as an end. Secretly, they are tired of life's struggles and are okay with this diagnosis as the final surrender. Sometimes the internal fire for life flickers low. If you are wavering, go to your heart to find and fan the embers that are still smoldering for life.

I heard a profound explanation of logic-based living (the left brain) versus heart-based living (the higher mind): our physical brain was never designed to solve difficult problems, create, or run the show. We have been taught to believe that the brain works in this way. We strain to come up with answers from the limited resources of the left brain, but it is solely the "workhorse." This modus operandi can be the source of our conundrums.

The theory espouses that the brain's job is to carry out what the higher mind asks of us, which, in essence, comes from the heart. All geniuses have told us that their most brilliant work did not come from analysis—it came from being in the zone; from allowing creativity to flow from "source" instead of chasing a solution. The heart/higher mind is where we can go to find our way on this fork in the road because it can see so much more. As Gary Zukav tells us in *The Seat of the Soul*, the personality is here to serve the energy of the soul. When we take our heart out of the equation, we leave valuable insights on the table.

Western culture is prone to ignoring the importance of the heart. It does far more than pump blood. Have you ever thought about the fact that the heart—the universal symbol of love and compassion—has a near immunity to cancer?

The HeartMath Institute is a non-profit organization that was founded in 1991. Doc Childre, Howard Marten, and their team have scientifically proven the intelligence and incredibly powerful frequencies of the heart. Their mission is to help bring people into physical, mental, and emotional coherence by harnessing the wisdom of the heart.

I was introduced to this information two decades ago and Heartmath's data is now widely recognized and accepted. There is a global shift back to what was known for thousands of years before the technological age—that the heart holds immeasurable genius and energy.

The heart speaks to us. If the voice is blaming, angry, or guilt-tripping, it is not the heart. Wounded thoughts and feelings are the ego at work. If the voice feels light and right, it is the heart. The home of our soul or spirit—wants the very best for us. Sometimes we hide from that voice or dismiss it altogether. My heart spoke to me first as a whisper, then a statement, next a shout, and finally a tsunami. The tsunami was another passage of breast cancer.

When pressed—like being in the gale of a cancer diagnosis—it is hard to let go and let the heart speak. We are given conflicting "facts" and viewpoints.

The day after I was hit by the tsunami, I instinctively started operating from my heart's intelligence out of a sense of self-preservation, instead of the decrees of logic, which is most often a voice filled with society's dogma, the good opinions, and the bullshit of others.

The quote from Charles Dickens *A Tale of Two Cities*, which I placed on the first page of this book has profound significance to me.

It was the best of times, it was the worst of times, it was the age of wisdom, it was the age of foolishness, it was the epoch of belief, it was the epoch of incredulity, it was the season of Light, it was the season of Darkness, it was the spring of hope, it was the winter of despair, we had everything before us, we had nothing before us, we were all going direct to Heaven, we were all going direct the other way. . . .

The grand paradox I mentioned in the blog post, *The Time of Your Life*, was that in the midst of my cancer journey, it was the worst time of my life juxtaposed with the best.

Yes, we need to incorporate logic. But more importantly, we need to go to our own inner knowing about what is the best for ourselves. Cancer asks you to step into your courage, a word derived from the French word, *coeur*—the heart. A human in cooperation with himself/herself is a symphony of the mind in service to the heart.

I admit that the road less traveled is a tough one. It has a lot of underbrush and rocks over which to maneuver and some serious peaks and valleys to traverse. You get bruised and scratched, and at times, find yourself exhausted and flattened from the strain. The beaten path is less menacing—of that there is no doubt—but the view and the beauty are not even remotely as grand and breathtaking.

Have you been living a juicy, passion-infused life or has it become hardened, like a calcified artery? Embrace the tenderness of your heart. Do not let the harshness, the craziness, and the pace of life destroy the beauty that lives inside of the most important part of you. Do not let cancer break your heart. Let it crack open, wider than ever before, and beat out a spectacular song of love, touching everyone in its sweet wake.

Article of interest:
Eat, Drink, Laugh
http://www.wandasthilaire.com/pdf/Eat%20Drink%20Laugh.pdf
(My après cancer celebration of life trip to Italy)

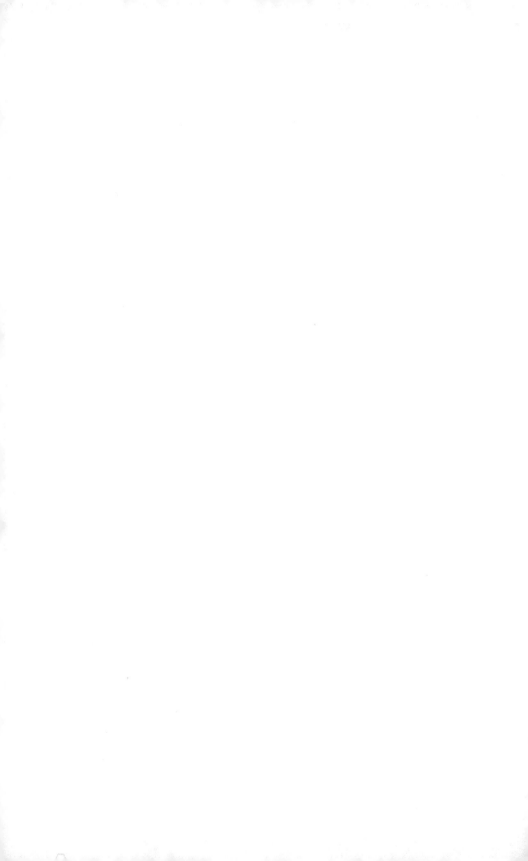

33

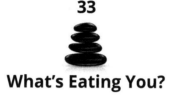

What's Eating You?

"When you hold onto your history, you do it at the expense of your destiny."
—Reverend T.D. Jakes

It's just you and me right now.

Can you be brutally honest and admit to whatever might be eating you?

There is an epidemic of illnesses in modern day society that appear to be untreatable, chronic, or incurable. We go to the doctor seeking cures and "bandage" fixes, but we seldom admit to the churning and tumultuous inner world we haul around on a daily basis. We do not reveal the old stories we are stuck in. Nor are we asked for them.

You may be living in a rat race of endless discontentment thinking it will never catch up to you, that one day you will fix the complications of your life, or that they will just work themselves out.

Is suffering a part of your daily existence?

Are you harboring deep resentments and hurts that are festering?

Unresolved trauma and sorrow sit in the body. Living a daily pattern of doubt and fear insidiously exhausts the immune system. Pay attention to how your body feels when you have strong emotions and negative thoughts; does it ache in a certain place, cause acid reflux, give you a migraine, or cause your back to spasm?

Are you tense all day long with a rollercoaster of varying emotional states?

I recently became aware of an interesting mental habit I harbor: my mind seeks problems to solve or things to be anxious about. If my life is in a state of equilibrium, my subconscious operating system will *still* look for something to mull over rather than just sink into the splendor of the moment—unless I consciously acquiesce.

Toxic mental patterns are clinically proven to be harmful to our health. Permitting unbridled moments of peace is a pattern that gives the human body breathing space to repair and rejuvenate.

If you are waiting for something in order to be happy, i.e. to get married, for a promotion, for more money, for a baby, for the resources to travel—you cause yourself unnecessary anxiety and will not enjoy the moment, as it is.

I have observed that many women diagnosed with breast cancer have perfectionist and/or self-judgmental tendencies. And what's more, we convince ourselves that it's justifiable. With this "time out" that we have been handed, we can cut ourselves slack and recognize that the pursuit of perfection is pointless.

Women with a propensity to put others first run the risk of burning out by refusing to nurture and care for themselves. We all need to be compassionate, gentle, and loving to ourselves first, so that we do not crash in the process of attending to everyone else's needs before our own.

My doctor told me of a patient with a diagnosis of breast cancer. She was rather proud of the fact that she and her husband had not had an argument or fight in twenty-five years of marriage. When the doctor asked her how that was possible, she admitted she was always afraid that if she spoke her mind, her husband would leave her.

After some post-cancer psychological therapy she decided to start asserting herself. She began to express her opinions and desires. At first her husband was taken aback, but as time went on he got used to her new ways. She felt a tremendous sense of freedom and relief. Twenty-five years of swallowing resentment and hurt and not speaking your truth is corrosive to your health.

Pre-cancer in 2010, an inner voice spoke to me and I did not listen because the message seemed irrational. It nagged at me, but I thought it was ridiculous. It pressed.

Quit your job and do something radical. Change your life.

I responded with an emphatic refusal.

I can't. Not yet. What will I do? How will I pay my bills? Where will I live?

Your soul's directives can be silenced by your willfulness, but you will eventually pay the piper. With the diagnosis, I was forced to look at making changes in my life, my beliefs, and my habits in ways I had previously been unwilling to entertain.

Do *you* have a small voice you are muzzling? Is there something in the back of your mind that you know you should do, yet seems wildly illogical? If so, listen. It may tell you to take radical action that appears absurd. All kinds of excuses, fierce opposition, and denial will rear up. But if that voice will not be silenced, pay attention.

Stand back and take an objective look at your life, as would a stranger who was asked to assess it. Examine it.

- Do you dread going to work or have combative or bullying colleagues or bosses?
- Are you overworked at home, on the job, or both?
- Do you allow yourself real vacations with no cellphone or email contact?
- Are you withering in an abusive, dead, or sexless relationship?
- Do you have any hobbies or side careers that allow your creative self to blossom, or is creativity a long-forgotten dream?
- Do you have a broken or closed heart that needs healing?
- Are you buried under a mountain of debt?
- Are you nursing old wounds and using them as an excuse to stay stuck?
- Are you overweight and justifying the absence of an exercise regime?
- Do you believe in a higher power and have a sense of connection to something other than what you can see or do you believe you are going it alone?
- Are you over-parenting and getting caught in dramas that you needn't be involved in?
- Are you always saying no to invitations, offers, or adventures?
- Is your life rigidly structured with no room for spontaneity?
- Are you engulfed in technology and social media overload?
- Do you live in a constant mode of competition?
- Do you allow yourself a good dose of pleasure each week or is your life a grind of chores, duties, and responsibility?
- Do you consistently make yourself wrong and feel like you're a "screw up?"
- Do you live in a clean and healthy environment or are you surrounded by chaos and clutter or toxicity in your home or workplace?
- Do you have an eating disorder or does your diet consist of a lot of fake and fast food?
- Are you lying to yourself or others?
- Is your vocabulary toxic and hostile?
- Do you live in the past?
- Do your children run your life?
- Are you chronically sleep deprived?

- Do you perpetually feel life is unfair and that you never get what you want—that your life is in a holding pattern or an endless waiting game?
- Do you know, deep down, that you are selling your soul for something?
- Do you feel your life is meaningless?
- Do you feel like you're an imposter in your career and that one day, you'll be "found out?"
- Do you have addictions that help to numb painful feelings?
- Are you pretending to be someone you are not and living a lie?
- Are you obsessing and perseverating about something or someone?
- Are you barely holding it together each day?
- Are you feigning ignorance about the impact of your negative actions or behavior on others?
- Do you keep a "catalogue" of every slight, each perceived insult, all things you consider offensive—a running list that you hold against others?
- Are you consumed with envy or jealousy?
- Do you blame the government, management, the establishment, or other people for your problems?
- Were/are you abused or are you an abuser?
- Are you resisting something important?
- Do you feel deep guilt for an infidelity or some wrong you feel you've done?
- Are you relentlessly trying to control everything?
- Do you have feelings of ineffectiveness or a lack of results in your life?
- Are you constantly fighting against something(s) or someone?

Be brutally honest. Are you chronically holding any of these emotional states on a regular basis?

- Anger
- Annoyance
- Anxiety
- Resentment
- Hurt
- Heartbreak
- Doubt
- Fear

- Guilt
- Grief
- Grudges
- Guardedness
- Paranoia
- Harsh judgment
- Self-righteousness
- Shame
- Self-loathing
- Disappointment
- Frustration
- Oppression
- Obsessiveness
- Regret
- Sadness
- Scarcity
- Hatred
- Suppression

The avoidance of painful memories and situations can cause us to self-medicate with substances, shopping, sex, workaholic tendencies, food, etc. If you are harboring a dark secret you find shameful, it will affect your wellbeing. If you carry a heavy cross of guilt, it will wear you down. Holding onto a hurt keeps you stuck.

The first step is to admit it to yourself. If you can discuss it with a professional, do so. If not, write it out in a private, well-hidden journal—all of it—and then burn it. If there is a wrong you feel you have done that can be made right, resolve it. These secrets are only one small aspect of life. They do *not* define us, nor are they meant to destroy us.

Sarah, a friend of a friend, recently passed away from cancer. She was not responding well to treatments and I asked if there was a deep hurt this lovely, gentle mother of three was carrying. My friend insisted there was no profound pain Sarah was withholding.

Sarah's best friend, Karen, came from overseas to be with her the last few weeks of her life. After she passed, Karen revealed that Sarah had endured a turbulent and violently abusive childhood, one that she had never mentioned to her close friends. After a divorce, her mother had essentially abandoned her when she married another man. Sarah always portrayed a quiet and peaceful demeanor, but hidden on the inside, she was suffering a long-standing pain. Pretending all is perfect when we are anguished has consequences.

In metaphysics, cancer is considered a response to a deep hurt or long-standing resentment or can be a buried secret eating away at the self. Reliving the painful past produces the same harmful chemicals in your system as though it is happening right *now*. It is a form of self-abuse. Now is the time to release repressed emotions and those 'forever' hurts. Now is the perfect moment to make peace with the past.

If you have trouble accepting a metaphysical perspective, from a conservative and medically acknowledged source, the Center for Disease Control cites that there is an emotional component to 85% of *all illnesses*. Further to that, new studies reveal that your viewpoint about the stress in your life is more important than the circumstances; if you believe what is happening is harmful to your health, it becomes so.

As previously stated, emotions and trauma get trapped in our physical bodies. Energy work such as Reiki, Acupressure, Biodynamic Craniosacral Therapy, Jin Shin Do, Shiatsu, Rolfing and Trager massage, EFT, The Emotion Code, and Reflexology can help release stuck emotional traumas.

In *My Stroke of Insight*, brain scientist Jill Bolte Taylor wrote eloquently about the fascinating experience she had during her stroke, which affected the left hemisphere of her brain. She emphatically explains that peace is just a thought away. We can choose to obsessively regurgitate our old hurts or we can opt to control our thoughts and stop re-stimulating the same emotional loops. She says all we need do is give our mind something else to think about—to choose a different trail. The quality of our thoughts dictates our happiness.

I recently reframed an old "mistake" that has haunted me and negatively impacted my life in many ways. I changed my perspective from seeing myself as having poor judgment— which resulted in a long-term lack of self-trust and an erosion of confidence—to realizing that my decision was based on good intentions, a sense of adventure, and was done in the name of love. I had the guts to take a chance on something many wouldn't. Those who fail frequently are those who dare greatly.

There is a beauty in life's paradox, one that we usually miss. When we are prepared to release that which we cling to so tightly—old wounds we keep alive, worn out relationships, jobs we abhor—when we let go, doors open in ways we had never imagined and miraculous healings can occur. Speak to your body and ask it to gently let go of the old pain and sad stories.

Change is not easy and human beings are often resistant to making different choices. And it is very difficult for us to own our dramas. But healing from something as serious as cancer requires some manner of transformation.

Facing and dealing with our secret inner world is the next frontier in medicine. One courageously important question to ask yourself and answer with raw honesty is: *What am I willing to change in order to heal?*

A side note for highly sensitive people:

I arrived into life thin-skinned. My childhood was tumultuous and I was confused by bad behavior. In school, bullies mystified me. Betrayals of friends and lovers have disturbed me to the core of my being. And I have never, ever understood the incredible violence of Earth. I have struggled with society's digression from freedom to ever tightening restriction and surveillance, and maybe you have too.

But I have found ways to pacify my sensitivity by honoring who I am in spite of the "norm." I never had children very purposefully. I have the soul of a gypsy and after I divorced, I didn't remarry. I refuse to participate in watching any violence, subjugation, or abuse. I come alive at night and am slow to wake in the mornings. I detest winter. I realized after cancer #2 that corporate life and all that went with it was not conducive to my true nature. I made a firm decision to never again work for organizations that don't match my values. And all of that is okay.

Duly note that sensitivity is, in essence, a belief. For instance, I believe violence is a form of insanity and that it deeply affects people's mindsets; therefore, I will never pay (or not pay) to watch it in any form. I could choose another point of view, but I don't want to. I prefer not to become desensitized to violence.

If you are highly sensitive, it is your right to live a gentle, slow life. Incorporating sensuality is a potent antidote to the harshness of the world. Beauty, nature, art, poetry, moving music, delectable whole food, and simplicity and order can soothe agitation caused by the dissonance. If you are uncomfortable following the herd, permit yourself to live in a way that best suits your biorhythms and emotional frequency.

TED Talks | How to make stress your friend
Kelly McGonigal
https://youtu.be/RcGyVTAoXEU

What if? ...

*"I said to my soul, be still and wait without hope, for hope would be hope
for the wrong thing; wait without love, for love would be love of the wrong
thing; there is yet faith, but the faith and the love are all in the waiting.
Wait without thought, for you are not ready for thought: So the darkness
shall be the light, and the stillness the dancing."*
—T.S. Eliot

After following Dr. Joe Dispenza's[1] work for the past few years, I made
a promise to myself that this year I would attend a workshop to hear
him speak—in the flesh—and participate in experiential exercises.
When I submitted my final flood insurance claim, I set the intention
that my drowned Barbie collection would make it so. Barbie came
through.

Last week I took a road trip with my mum to the Okanagan, picked
up my sister—a reluctant participant—and then drove on to the lushness
of spring in Vancouver for the workshop.

I was thrilled when midway through the first morning, I saw the
AH-HA spark of understanding hit my sister. For Christmas I had given
her the book *Breaking the Habit of Being Yourself*, along with two meditation CDs. I knew she had not opened either of them. Beforehand she
had argued the reasons she could not attend the workshop and only
after I gave up trying to convince her did she yield. I actually saw the
moment she grasped how this philosophy could work to greatly improve
the quality of her life.

In my life, I am long overdue to break the habit of being myself.
Neither I, nor Dr. Joe, are implying that we are not good enough as we
are. His life's mission is to show us how to get back to our peaceful and
powerful essence, the one we came in with before life happened.

What he teaches us is how to gently transform the layers of our past
troubles into wisdom and begin to create a new future that has nothing
to do with our old history.

---

1   http://www.drjoedispenza.com/

We develop beliefs and habits based on our environment and circumstances. Our self-talk can become something so insidious and seductive that we do not even realize the harmful stories we have been telling ourselves, sometimes for decades.

In the modern world, a vast array of addictions are rising at startling rates. A recovering heroin addict, Russell Brand, spoke eloquently on Oprah about the nature of addiction. He nailed it when he said that it is the desperate longing to escape from our emotions that send us into the arms of an awaiting temptress of choice.

Most addictions are obvious: alcohol, drugs, gambling, cigarettes, porn, food, etc. A well-kept secret is that the compulsive and obsessive emotional states we harbor are just as addictive. Ever burgeoning scientific research now exposes how the chemicals of negative feelings such as anger, resentment, fear, and unworthiness operate in the same way as an addiction to cocaine.

The incoherence in the body, the mind, and the heart makes us reach for something to ease the discomfort and discordance. If left unchecked for too long, this disharmony can create disease and chaos.

Thankfully I do not have an addictive nature when it comes to mind-altering substances. Although I am a student of personal growth and the philosophical, I had yet to find an instrument for lasting change, one that can appease the lure of oscillating emotional states—my addiction of "choice."

An addiction is something that you cannot stop. If you are honest with yourself, what in your life might you be addicted to?

With the new science of neuroplasticity—the science that a brain can fundamentally and permanently change—we are empowered in ways previously considered impossible.

Is it easy? I would say that vigilance is the key, and that desire and dedication to change is imperative.

So how do we do it?

First and foremost, with time spent in meditation. A brain in constant analysis or high alert mode is not a coherent brain. We have all read or been told about the benefits of meditation, but do you know how exponentially transformative the effects are through daily practice? I didn't.

Prior to the workshop, I tried the recommended meditations and my inner whirling dervish kicked and bucked like a wild bronco. My analytical side did not have enough personal evidence to inspire or motivate me to continue and my body cunningly convinced me not to bother.

I discovered that what lies underneath our jumping thoughts and pinball-like worry is not only our aching and yearning, but also our truth. On the other side of our churning discontentment lies peace. In the power of the present, we can create a new future.

What I love about this work is that it aligns with my deepest wish to help people change tracks *before* the train hits them. We are often motivated to change after the diagnosis, or bankruptcy, or accident, or divorce. But why not before, while life is giving us gentle signs and messages that we are off course? Ennui, despair, resentment, dysfunctional relationships, seething anger, anxiety, sleeplessness, jobs we hate, or weird new health conditions are all signs that something is amiss.

If you think this is all too dry or not worth the effort, au contraire *mon frere*. Dr. Joe had us do one of the rehearsals (like visualization) for something playful and fun; he is a strong proponent of using these tools for light and joyful happenstances.

In one meditation in Vancouver I imagined that a man (or men) would flirt; the evidence would be that one such man would buy me a drink. The next evening my sister and I ate at a buzzing tiny Greek restaurant on Robson. The craggy Greek man at the door lit up and insisted we wait out the line. He was eager for us to stay, so we did. Inside, he bought us both a generous shot of ouzo and his son stopped to tell us that the old man was the original owner and intimated that it was an unusual honor for him to make such a gesture. Five minutes later, I realized the ouzo was my drink—and that I didn't specify *hot* guy! The servers were warm and friendly and spent a lot of time chatting with us. My sister's playful visualization came through a day later—it had to do with a "Greek god" nudge, nudge, wink, wink. It was the fun side of the inner-work and a great motivator to continue.

Over 200 people attended the workshop, most with a profound commitment to bring about freedom within to create change without. I believe most left with renewed hope and all left with a ladder to climb out of whatever pit, shallow or deep, that they want to rise above.

What if ... we all made quiet meditation each day a priority in order to heal our inner worlds instead of allowing our outer worlds to dictate our states of mind?

What if ... the great paradox is that if we could fall in love with life and with ourselves first before we see our dreams show up—and live in gratitude—we could find a little slice of heaven while on Earth?

What if ... this is the science behind what Jesus and Buddha taught?

And what if ... planet Earth could hit the tipping point for peace by individuals letting go of their past pains and old grievances with fervor and devotion to become a light for others to follow?

In my quest to live my life by heart and inspire others to do the same, I am grateful to have had the opportunity to spend time learning how to cultivate grace. I pray to be stronger than my history, to rise above my demons, and to be the miracle I seek.

And I pray the same for you.

What if? ...
http://wp.me/p2ACw4-od
lifebyheart.wandasthilaire.com

34

Forgive

"Resentment is like drinking poison and then hoping it will kill your enemies."
—Nelson Mandela

When we visit a doctor for a serious illness, the topic of forgiveness is never discussed. But it should be. I have studied volumes on the healing power of forgiveness and about the dramatic destruction that stems from the lack of forgiveness.

When the subject of forgiveness comes up, oftentimes people brush off the idea; they believe they have nobody and nothing to forgive. I implore you to genuinely consider where a lack of forgiveness may linger in your life. Become conscious of anything you have stuffed away in your unconscious, maybe from many years ago.

There is a high cost to hatred. Dr. Alex Lloyd, author and founder of *The Healing Codes*, says that in all of the years he has lectured and counseled people, he has never seen a significant health problem where a lack of forgiveness was not an issue. He met Dr. Ben Johnson, a doctor who lectures all over the world about cancer and Dr. Johnson concurred that he has found a correlation between cancer and a lack of forgiveness.

In *The Dynamic Laws of Healing*, Catherine Ponder states: "*It is an immutable mental and spiritual law that when there is a health problem, there is a forgiveness problem. You must forgive if you want to be permanently healed.*" That is one powerful and sweeping statement, yet I have repeatedly read similar declarations in my studies. This concept is an opinion—one you can consider or disregard—but if it angers you, ask yourself why?

Anxiety, hatred, and resentment facilitate disease by flat-lining the immune system. Adrenaline and cortisol, the chemicals of survival, race through our system, seeking the enemy and shutting down natural killer cells which fight disease. The enemy is all in our minds—our repetitive thoughts and our capricious emotions.

Too often, we wallow in the past. We relive the wrongs that were done to us, or we foster our hurts. We take things personally. We harbor grudges and vendettas over a single sentence someone once said. We are too proud to make peace by extending the "olive branch."

My ex used the phrase, "I don't get mad; I get even." Revenge never, ever works out in your best interest. A lack of forgiveness is poisonous and vengefulness is like adding fuel to an already caustic fire within. As poet, artist, and philosopher, Kahlil Gibran, said, "An eye for an eye, and the whole world would be blind."

One thing we need to keep in mind about human nature is that if people know better, they usually do better. Someone may have wronged us due to a difficult period in his or her secret life or for some reason that we know nothing about. Oftentimes it is not personal. (*Hanlon's razor is an aphorism expressed in various ways including "Never attribute to malice that which is adequately explained by stupidity."* —Wikipedia.) We all make bad choices at one time or another that are not specifically out of maliciousness.

I cannot forgive him/her; I just can't do it, is a common avowal. Forgiving someone does not mean you continue to remain in an abusive situation. You do not have to reconnect to forgive. And it does not indicate that you condone the poor behavior of another. It signifies the clearing of your heart and mind from the malaise of resentment. It means that you forgive for your own wellbeing. Forgiveness releases you from an internal prison—you do it for you. You can walk away from someone because they are no longer a constructive influence, but you can do so with forgiveness. Holding onto self-righteousness equals pain. Remember, we are all imperfect.

Bad memories reemerge so that you can embrace the opportunity to heal them. By applying forgiveness to past transgressors, you return yourself to the power of the present moment rather than living in the past.

I still do not understand why it is so difficult to forgive oneself, but for me, this has been my Mount Everest. I believe others are forgivable, yet I still must consciously work to relinquish harsh judgments about my perceived failures. We cannot always retract the foolish things we have done or undo poor choices, but we can forgive ourselves for them.

Huge guilt issues and self-recrimination may crop up with cancer patients if one has smoked, used recreational drugs, or participated in other harmful activities. Self-acceptance and forgiveness for our personal lapses is essential. With cancer it is critical that we forgive *ourselves*. And yes, you, dear one, (and I) deserve forgiveness.

An effective way to open your heart and heal is to systematically think of everyone who remains a source of un-forgiveness in your life, then apply proclamations of forgiveness. You can list everyone who you feel has hurt you back from childhood onward: every family member, every boss, every teacher, every coworker, every friend, every boyfriend/girl-friend—everyone, including yourself. Even God.

It may sound like a daunting task, but in a relaxed state, your mind will supply you with recollections. Give yourself permission to heal the past. You can work through this with a qualified therapist, pastor, or some type of healing professional.

A forgiveness ceremony can be powerful. Write down everyone you are ready to forgive and burn the paper, drown it in water, tear it up, or send it off in a bottle. You may have held a lack of forgiveness for many years and, if so, it would behoove you to make a declaration of forgiveness each night until you feel it is resolved.

A friend of mine took her mother, who had cancer, to a mountain chalet for a weeklong getaway. She asked her mother to write a letter each day. Firstly, to her own mother and father about any and all of her grudges, hurts, betrayals, or resentments and then seal it in an envelope and set it by the fireplace. The next day, she wrote a letter to her siblings. The next day, her children. The following day, her friends and extended family. Then, her husband. The sixth day, old loves. The last day, any colleagues or random people she felt had hurt her. On the final day, they burned all of the sealed envelopes in the fire. It was an extremely cathartic process for her mum.

EFT tapping, as outlined in chapter 28, is also a wonderful technique to use in letting go of grievances and forgiving others. You can go over your list to tap out the resentments and tap in the forgiveness. EFT practitioners are available to help personalize a program and lead you to clemency.

Years ago I learned of another simple method that can be modified as a forgiveness exercise from the book *The Heartmath Solution*. It is surpris-ingly powerful and takes only 5 minutes a day to do (until you feel that you are clear from resentments). HeartMath teaches how to regulate emotional states and take responsibility for how we feel and behave. We regain our personal power and come to understand that another cannot hurt us unless we allow them to.

Get into a relaxed position in a quiet place. Drop into your heart by thinking of something or someone you love or appreciate dearly. Place your attention on your heart. You may feel it flutter or become warm.

Imagine breathing through your heart and stay steady in your focus on the heart center. Then send intentions of love, blessings, appreciation, goodwill, and most importantly, forgiveness to the transgressor.

When you feel someone has done something horrible to you this can be a difficult concept to wrap your head around. Why should I bless a boss who stole a big commission from me? You want me to send appreciation to my jerk of an ex? Why would I send love to the landlord who is rude and never repairs anything?

Why? Because amazing things happen as a consequence of this practice. At first it can be challenging, but soon you feel yourself soften. Your fury dissipates. You start seeing the person in a new light; you remind yourself that they may be hurt or broken, and could be suffering too. You will discover that thinking of their trespasses no longer holds the negative charge that it did before. I have experienced amazing breakthroughs in relationships using this technique. But more importantly, I have been set free from resentments, hurt, and anger. And there is nothing like the feeling of a mind free of internal disputes.

In a Master Class, Oprah spoke about one of her infamous AH-HA moments that occurred during an old show. One of her guests explained that forgiveness meant giving up the hope that the past could be any different than it was and accepting that an event happened as it did. She called it a "transcendent" moment that changed her and she said that she no longer holds grudges.

A lack of forgiveness is one of the most venomous toxins on the planet. All we need do is turn on the news to see just how brutally destructive it is. When you forgive, you grant yourself a massive opportunity to heal. It is an act of self-compassion that is more monumental in altering your life to the good than you may have ever considered. You will lighten your mind, your body, and your life by dropping a heavy backpack that you did not even know you were carrying.

Forgiveness is the ultimate act of grace and can be a game changer that can heal things you would not have thought possible. It does not change the past, but it does change the future.

Imagine what the world would be like if we all forgave each other.

35

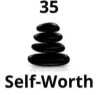

Self-Worth

The lilies whispered, "You accept far less than you deserve.
And when you settle for less than you deserve, you receive an
even further diminished version of what you accept."
—Wanda St. Hilaire
The Cuban Chronicles

The worth of your precious self has no correlation to a diagnosis of cancer. Nor is it what you do, the amount of money you make, how much you weigh, how attractive you are, your marital status, the opulence of your home, or the brand name on your possessions.

Nothing will tear down your morale and self-esteem faster than comparing yourself to others. Competing with the Joneses is an endless and futile pursuit. My personal odyssey has absolutely no parallel to my neighbor's. Outward appearances are illusory and constantly alter; self-worth needs to be an inside job that remains solid and does not elevate or sink with circumstances or perceived failures. It also should not depend on the good opinion or approval of others. I struggle to keep myself from comparing where I am in relation to people in my circle. When I get caught in the notion of disparity, I remind myself that I did not come here to be anyone else or live another's path, and neither did you.

We have all seen, in the fantasyland of fame, how image and money matters not when it comes to self-worth. The news is filled with musicians and actors who appear to have it all, yet die from "accidental" overdose or suicide—the deepest form of unhappiness there is. When our state of affairs feels unbearable or the world is not giving us the feedback we'd hoped for, it can be hard to hold strong. This is when we need to remember that our outer shell is only temporary and that our spirit is the bedrock of who and what we really are.

Oftentimes we keep how little we are accepting in life a well-hidden secret. We may fume while we silently tolerate a cheapskate partner who is not carrying their weight in the cost of living. We could begrudgingly accept a salary that is well below our level of expertise. We might be enduring a serious lack of respect from our children. Or playing mute in a subtly abusive relationship.

We can feel victimized by people, but the truth is, it is we who set the stage; it is we who teach others how to treat us and show people how little we will accept. As Eleanor Roosevelt once said, "No one can make you feel inferior without your consent." Accepting the crumbs at the bottom of the pan is insidious and is indicative of our level of self-worth. It wears us down until we feel small and insignificant. It makes us irritable. It definitely affects our wellbeing and can ultimately affect our health.

The measure of what is good or bad, beautiful or homely, rich or poor, is highly subjective and relative. If you had been born into the Masai tribe you would pierce your earlobes and elongate them by wearing elephant tusks as a symbol of beauty. In Mauritius, the fatter the woman, the more desirable as a wife. Believe it or not, wearing a rhinoplasty bandage is considered a status symbol in Iran. In North America, all we need do is look through airbrushed and manipulated images in magazines to see the falsified and unattainable norms. Prevailing standards are arbitrary and an invention of every culture. Further to that, they morph from year to year, and evolve from era to era.

Unfortunately, Western society places an absurdly high value on image and outward appearances of perfection (which does not exist). I recently worked an event for a friend in a mall setting and we were located in front of a brand name designer store. This shop sells women's bags and accessories that are essentially *plastic* and are manufactured at the same place as Walmart bags. Because of the metal logo, the value is unfathomably inflated. Women swarmed the outlet and filed out in droves with their shopping bags brimming with purchases. It saddened me. It is only the label that makes these products so sought after—all because it gives us a feeling of status, which is a bogus sense of self-worth. The world is a rapidly changing place, so invent your own rules and build your self-worth based on your inner awesomeness, not by distorted standards set by fools.

We can have robust self-esteem; we may know what our talents and skills and redeeming qualities are, yet in the deeper recesses, still have little self-worth. What does this have to do with cancer? Everything.

When the harmful chemicals of self-dislike (and especially self-loathing) course through your body on a daily basis, you hinder your healing. A solid sense of self-worth is another piece of the puzzle in wellbeing.

Your intrinsic value is as unique as each snowflake that lands on the planet. You are an integral piece of life. You *"are"* and do not require a "rating." You are worthy of love and have every right to experience a sense of belonging because you are a vital part of life. You deserve to live.

Never forget: *You matter.*

Let it Go

"Cry. Forgive. Learn. Move on. Let your tears water the seeds of your future happiness."
—Steve Maraboli

A few weeks ago I completed an assignment to review with my life coach. Before we met, I added something to my intentions for 2016. With deep deliberation, I wrote down a list of what I am willing to let go of this year. The list was only six points long, but it was monumental.

Two days after I made that declaration to the field of life, poo hit the fan. In the span of a week, some serious letting go happened at mind-dizzying speed. I should have specified: *gently and with ease.* I didn't really mean, let's get rid of it all in the next *week*.

Even when we know something or someone is not working out for the best, it is not always easy to let go. We cling. We hang onto relationships that are toxic or past their due date. We stay at jobs that we hate. We hold onto old clothes we will never wear. We even keep stale food tucked away in cupboards or layered under ice in our freezers.

Why?

Fear of the unknown.

My mum has a belief which is evident in a saying she has repeated for years: Better the devil you know that the one you don't. In other words, she would rather deal with an arse she knows than someone she does not. The next one could be worse.

Scarcity.

What if there is nothing past this? What if I can't find another job? What if I never know love before I die? What if ... *this* is as good as it gets?

Not wanting to deal with confrontation.

Oh God, it will be a mess. I'll have to confront the situation or person and I don't need more problems in my life. What if I just let it ride? What if I just accept things as they are and carry on?

Misguided notions of strength and stoicism.

I am not the type to give up. I will see it through to the end. I'm rough, tough, and used to hardships. This may just be my lot in life.

Playing small.

I don't have to step up my game in this relationship, job, friendship. I can cruise if I stay and keep things status quo. This is so much easier than going for gold.

Loss of identity.

Who will I be without him/her? Who will I be without this career? This job? What will I do with my time?

The vacuum that precedes the change.

After the letting go comes the hollow hell phase. I do not want to face that. I cannot face that. I will *lose* it.

Sometimes we are given lessons, which repeat over and over until we seize the opportunity to step up, take a stand, and let go. A few weeks ago, a repeating theme showed up in my life (oh, joy). An unforeseen challenge roused a tremendous physical response in my body. It also triggered a flashback to a strikingly similar moment.

I remembered sitting across from my young boss in a busy café. He had just told me that he had been on a "covert" mission and had visited my accounts, something I already knew because my annoyed clients had told me. He shared his findings, which seemed to perplex and almost disappoint him.

"I can't believe it, but they all love you. I didn't get one bad comment, one negative shred of feedback," he said.

"Yes, I know." (It wasn't my first rodeo. I had once been accused by another manager of *paying* my clients to say wonderful things about me—as though they could not possibly be true.)

I have decades of sales experience and my forte is relationship building, which this young man had yet to conceive the value of. This was in the midst of an economic crash and while my competitors were struggling with 50% decreases in sales, I was sitting at a mere 6% deficit.

He went on to tell me a long story about the new equipment the company was buying and their plan (and costs) for offering better service. And then he proceeded to cut my base wage in half, combined with a new cockamamie commission plan. Stunned, I recalled my very first thought: *Tell him to F off. Shake his hand, tell him to F off, and then walk away.*

But I didn't.

I did not want to have to search for another job. I did not want to retrain. I unequivocally did not want to kiss more managerial butt. I was in fear for my survival. So I stayed. And I allowed myself to feel that my worth, my many years of expertise, had been swiftly sliced into half of its value.

Every day, I awoke unhappy because of this lack of respect and devaluation. I still gave my clients the best of me because I cared for them, but I felt a deep resentment as I struggled to cover my basic needs. I allowed two young, inexperienced managers to determine *my* sense of self-worth. And within six months, I was diagnosed with cancer—after a 20-year long triumph.

This time, I saw the writing on the wall. I had just been emphatically praised and had been doing an impeccable job at a demanding and unusual part-time contract. I had gone above and beyond. And in one shocking moment, I was undervalued in a way that defied all ethics and logic. This time I recognized that same repeating lesson; I finally got it. In spite of the suffocating scarcity loop, and in spite of my long-standing pattern of settling for a lack of appreciation with a stiff upper lip, I let go. I did not engage in any drama. I walked away.

I could almost see my spirit guides high-fiving and doing Pharrell's *Happy* dance, interspersed with shouts of "hallelujah!" and "at last!"

There begs the question: was it a good thing or a bad thing? My normal response would be "bad." But by shifting to neutrality, I can see the gift behind the opportunity to take a stand for myself. I don't know what follows, but I do know that from my soul's perspective, it's a good thing. That event created a domino effect. If you know anything about tarot, it's been like living in The Tower card (disaster, upheaval, sudden change, revelation).

For most of us, there is great discomfort in letting go of what we know. Before the new arrives, there is a deafening emptiness. This, my friends, is the tough spot. This is the space of nothingness where the flotsam is behind you in the wake and land cannot be seen ahead.

The challenge is to find peace in the void. To not fall prey to bobbing around in the boat of life waiting for the sharks in a state of hopelessness. To muster optimism even though you see no evidence of a shoreline. To embrace the uncertainty.

The strength and courage is in the letting go of things we know are dishonoring to the self. The point of power is in the paradox; in order to have what we deeply desire, we must let go of our attachments to circumstances and relationships that are blocking the path to our 'right' life.

What's on the other side of the abyss? We cannot know. Could be good, could be bad. Or … it may possibly be something bigger, better, and more bodacious than we could ever imagine.

Be brave.
Be bold.
Let it go.

Let it Go
http://wp.me/p2ACw4-xt
lifebyheart.wandasthilaire.com

36

To Thine Own Self be True

"When one is pretending the entire body revolts."
—Anaïs Nin

In Anita Moorjani's[1] book, *Dying to be Me*, she shares her most profound lesson in a near-death cancer experience. When she slipped into a coma, she saw how she had spent her entire life trying to please others, and had unhappily followed a multitude of ludicrous and conflicting rules and cultural mores. She had kept herself in check through fear and had always put on a happy face contrary to her true feelings. She learned that we come here to be exactly who we are and that self-love, self-acceptance, and complete authenticity is the name of the game on Earth's playing field.

Here is a defining question: *are you living a life that is being true to you?*

One of the most misery-generating things you can do is pretend to be something you are not or live by someone else's expectations and rules for life. It takes an inordinate amount of energy and strain to be something other than who you are. The guilt of feeling you have not met another's standards damages your body and diminishes your quality of life.

If you have any inkling (or glaring alarms) that you are not living your truth, contemplate the reasons why. After you are through the initial thick of this journey, if you are not living a life that is authentic, what will you do to change it? There is tremendous relief when you drop any false pretenses or masks and allow yourself honest self-expression.

I discovered that in a weird twist, cancer gets you off the hook—a hook you should not have been hanging from in the first place. People more readily accept your choices when you remind them that you have had a brush with your mortality and want to live a life true to yourself.

Big things may need to be altered and that can be a daunting task. There may be people who do not want you to change. But you are not here to

---

1   http://anitamoorjani.com/

make others more comfortable by being whom and what they want you to be. You are here to be 100% *you* as you were uniquely and preciously created, with all of your predilections, desires, and character quirks.

I know people who refuse to be whom and what they are. Some live contrary to what they know in their heart is best for their overall health and happiness because *someone else* will not approve. Others live life like a marathon when their natural rhythm is that of a tortoise. Some wear clothing that has nothing to do with their personality because it is the acceptable norm amongst their peers. And some are constantly monitoring themselves by the benchmark of another's decree.

Many years ago, a good friend of mine married young. Her husband was handsome and extremely artistic. Their home was impeccable and stylish. Almost all of his friends were gay and I suspected that he was too. They divorced after a few years and he moved on to a relationship with another woman.

One day we got a call that he was missing. Groups of friends went out searching for him. Unfortunately, he chose to end his life instead of come out in his truth. He was a talented, fine man and the world needed him. But he could not allow himself liberation from the false identity he had created because of his assumptions of how his conservative family would react. This is the ultimate toll of squelching who you are, but illness can also be a symptom of living behind a fake guise.

Are you a non-conformist living a mal-adapted life? Sometimes we live in a box of self-imposed rules without realizing the stifling limitations we have placed on ourselves. We may set perfectionism as the bar to aspire to when all we really want to do is chill and enjoy life. None of us need be perfect in such an imperfect world.

Living in your true frequency—the culture, the climate, rural or city, or even the country you live in—is important to flourishing authentically. I was born on the flatlands in a December's freezing winter, but I no more suit snow and a conservative prairie life than I do living on Pluto. It is not that I think a typical Canadian lifestyle is wrong, it is that it it's simply not ideal for *me*.

I have a friend who was living in a large American city when she went on vacation to Mexico. She knew instantly it was the right place for her. In spite of having a good job centered on her degree, she moved twenty-some years ago, built a business, and started a family there. Even during tough times she has never considered moving back to the USA. Sometimes we need to transplant ourselves in order to live optimally, even if makes no sense to others.

If there is only one thing you impart from this book, I hope it is the message that "being you" is what you came here for. You, as much as anyone on Earth, have the right to speak your truth. You deserve to live the lifestyle that best suits you. Give yourself consent to be true to your purpose, whether it be a gardener or a politician, a burlesque dancer or a judge. What comes naturally to you is your exquisite gift to the world. If someone does not approve of you—no matter their importance—so what? As I have heard Oprah say, you cannot live a brave life without disappointing someone.

Laugh when you feel like laughing (roll on the floor if you must) and cry when you need to cry. Do not dampen your innate expression to impress others. Do not stuff your emotions or feelings, your desires and needs for *anyone*. I implore you to give yourself permission to be the original, one-of-a-kind you, no matter whom or what you are. The world needs your incomparable stamp on it.

In his phenomenal commencement speech, Jim Carrey said: *So many of us choose our path out of fear disguised as practicality. What we really want seems impossibly out of reach and ridiculous to expect, so we never dare to ask the Universe for it.* (Read/watch here[1]—a thought-provoking discourse.)

Remember, if there were no crazy or weird people, we would have no airplanes or iPhones. There would be no Princes or Julia Childs or Jim Carreys gracing the world with their idiosyncratic brilliance. Non-conformity takes guts, but you have the strength and courage within you to live authentically.

People die with an inimitable song still unsung. They die because of the pain and grief for that sweet song.

Do not let that be you.

Sing.

---

1   https://tinyurl.com/k2tcdnj

A Dolphin in the Snow
03/9/13

"It gives me great pleasure indeed to see the stubbornness of an incorrigible nonconformist warmly acclaimed."
—Albert Einstein
(Me too, Mr. Einstein, me too.)

Authenticity is at the core of living life by heart. The heart does not operate by logic and it wants you to honor who you really are and to be completely who you came here to be. Without apology.

I *love* stories and my favorite ones are of people or animals overcoming incredible odds, underdogs succeeding, and people who have made radical reinventions. The other day, on Oprah Radio, I listened to a man who had been a successful lawyer speak with incredible passion about starting a mustard museum (say what?) much to his Jewish mother's mortification.

Our genuine selves are sometimes so deeply buried we don't have a clue who we are "not being" and what we are not doing. The whispers of the heart are easily drowned out by the staccato of life.

I have been excavating my inner world for years and thought that I was fairly cognizant of my true self. But going deeper (in the meditations of the emotional rehab I wrote of in an earlier post, *The Rabbit Hole of Reinventing Yourself*, Feb 5, 2013) it came to me that there may be even more layers to unearth to get to the real McCoy.

With a new onslaught of spring storms and exhausting hot flashes, I found myself unable to get out of my robe on Saturday—the best day of the frigging week. Uncharacteristically (especially since I get my coffee on the outside), I had no desire to leave the house or do anything more than read. Finally, at 8:00 pm, I showered and got dressed with only one mission in mind: go to McDonald's. For anyone who knows me, you'll read this as a Code Red Alert. Not only did I have a manic urge for McDonald's, I drove in and asked for the 'Depression Combo Pack.'

"What is that?" asked the cashier.

"A Big Mac, fries, *and* a hot fudge sundae," I said, and then gunned the car to get the goods.

"Having a bad day?" asked the young guy at the window with a sympathetic smile.

"*Yes.* I have never ordered $10 worth of McDonald's food in my life! And you can name that combo pack after me if you want."

The next day, when I awoke to a raging blizzard, I could have cleaned the snow off the sidewalks in a Bugs Bunny nanosecond; I was a Tasmanian devil of annoyance and white fury. (Unfortunately, Dispenza[1] does not lie when he says you have to lose your mind to redesign a new one.)

Why such agitation? I can tell you best in an analogous story that may trigger some insight into your own Tasmanian moments.

Let's imagine that the Earth is, by and large, Rabbit World. There's nothing implicitly wrong with rabbit life and there are billions of rabbits happily mating, reaching pinnacles in their careers, and living in gorgeous rabbit homes.

I have lived as a rabbit for most of my life. I was born into a rabbit family, went to rabbit schools, ate rabbit food, married a rabbit man—once upon a time, and have worked at many rabbit jobs. Most of those whom I love are rabbit people.

But, I am a dolphin. And I have lived much of my life with the notion that wanting to be my dolphin self is wrong and that I should try my very best to be a rabbit. The tenacity with which I've clung to that undertaking is rather mind-boggling. What has kept me going are the moments I've spent in a dolphin's life—I know it exists—and it is magnificent.

In Dolphin World[2], femininity is revered. Male dolphins act like males and female dolphins act like females. It is all very natural. When I date the rabbits, they are suspicious because they think nobody honestly wants to play that much and that I must have a hidden agenda.

I am given carrots, but dream of little, brightly colored fish. I find getting the carrots difficult. In the sea, abundance is everywhere, all of the time. There is an endless supply of whatever you need and it all flows effortlessly. Here, I have to live in the snow and dig deep for the carrots. Dolphins don't swim or breathe well in snow.

1 http://lifebyheart.wandasthilaire.com/creating-your-reality/
the-rabbit-hole-of-reinventing-yourself/
2 https://youtu.be/9bKwRW0l-Qk

Each day, I wake up as though I have been back to the sea in my sleep and I need to talk myself into rabbit life. I awaken reluctantly and drag myself out of my bed. Gradually, I succumb to rabbit life and its demands, although, as a dolphin, I frequently wonder why anyone would want to be a rabbit.

I am fascinated by all non-rabbits, ones like Laird Hamilton, Jane Goodall, Diane Fossey, and Ernest Hemingway. I have a few non-rabbit friends who have successfully defected to their rightful domains. I am sometimes happy for them and sometimes, ashamedly, green-gilled with envy.

I have played by rabbit rules. I have answered my whole life to boss rabbits who have frequently asked me if I was hitting the customer rabbits on the head with a hammer to get them to buy things.

Instead, I told the customer rabbits dolphin tales and brought them dolphin treats and gave them TLC. I know they liked this so much more than getting hit on the head with a hammer and that they were loyal because they liked my dolphin energy. But I always held an underlying fear that the boss rabbits would find out that I am a dolphin and would take away the carrots.

I am told I have to do many strange things in order to be successful in Rabbit World. I do as many as I can, but I am not "successful" by rabbit standards. Personally, I think swimming and telling dolphins stories and just being a dolphin *is* the definition of success.

When I went through cancer two, I made decisions from my dolphin self. I decided not to run back to my old job and old world, which would have nicely kept me at status quo in Rabbit Land. I innately knew it would be death for me. I chose to use the rabbit money I had painstakingly saved to recover in a dolphin's best environment.

I went to the ocean for six months and I lived life at its finest. Boisterous dolphins surrounded me. I ate dolphin food and I did dolphin things; walking on the beach, watching sunsets and full moons over the ocean, dancing, listening to foreign music in the streets each day. I often went on the ocean to bond with sea life, my hair blowing, the ocean mist and sun on my skin, the whales breaching, the manta rays floating by and … the dolphins[1] jumping out to say hello to a sister. I was in awe of life.

I lived in a dolphin house for the *very* first time in my life; a spectac-

1 https://youtu.be/9bKwRW0l-Qk

ular view of the sea on a hilltop; a cozy kitchen for cooking; a minimalist home with massive windows and a constant cool breeze blowing; a huge patio with a hammock and high power binoculars to see the craters on the moon at night; and a big bed I awakened in every morning with a view of the ocean. Every single day I gave thanks for being in Dolphin World.

I wrote my dolphin tales at an outdoor café in front of the ocean where both non-rabbits and rabbits came by to talk to me and visit. I sang in my new abode because, at last, I was inspired to sing once again.

I was so much in my frequency that the skin condition which had taken over my body and flared up to the extreme during treatments began to subside in one month. By the time I left, my skin was its smooth, clear self for the first time in eight years. (When I came back, the spots returned within one month).

I returned at ground zero financially, but with a bunch of dolphin ideas of how I would sustain my dolphin life and I was excited and optimistic. But the ideas didn't fly with the rabbits. I kept creating and trying. I went to rabbit school for six months to learn the "right" ways to make the plan work. And as time crept on, little-by-little, I built a trap of rabbit debt to survive.

In the process of trying to rewire my emotions, I see the crux of my angst is the confining trap I have created for myself in Rabbit World. How do you leave rabbit life to live the life you were born for from a trap of your own creation? There are likely 1000 solutions in Universal Mind, but from the cage, I can't see them.

Trying to create a dolphin's life by rabbit rules doesn't work. When you've wedged yourself on a fence keeping one foot firmly planted in Rabbit World and one dipping your toes back and forth in dolphin waters, it makes for a very irritating pain in the ass.

When we live out of sync with who we truly are and what we need for much too long, that's likely the place where we hit the wall.

Who are you not being?

What do you want that you tuck away as a one-day thing?

What things ignite a fire inside you that you ignore?

Here is a brilliant story from über unique non-rabbit, Amanda Palmer: The Art of Asking[1]. It is a tale of a woman who lives life by her own

---

1   https://youtu.be/xMj_P_6H69g

wildly nonconformist terms with an extraordinary trust in life, in the goodness of people, and in her art. What happened because she honored her "non-rabbitness" in a rabbit-dominant world, in spite of criticism and harassment, will astound you. It's 14 minutes of your life worth spending on a story that may shed a sliver of light on your own authentic and unique raison d'être.

The Dolphin in the Snow
http://wp.me/p2ACw4-er
lifebyheart.wandasthilaire.com

37

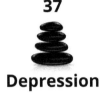

Depression

A tiny light
far out in the swells of the sea
and suddenly
a wave decimating it

Wait for it
Count on it
It will return
It wants to find you
—Wanda St. Hilaire
Of Love, Life and Journeys

Life can go from pulsing color to a bleak grey overnight with a diagnosis. The grief that washes over your life with cancer pulls at the light within. It darkens with its melancholic shadow. A diagnosis can deliver as much trauma as a severe car accident or a plundering tornado. When cancer follows on the heels of a misfortune, it can pack a punch. When it comes after a long series of disappointments and adversity, as it did for me, it can be devastating. It is okay to feel whatever you feel about the appearance of the C word in your life. Grief and depression may be another aspect of the journey.

When you are faced with daily reminders at the hospital or treatment center and are surrounded by people who appear emaciated and ill—and have the same disease—it is hard to focus on what you do want: 100% health, rather than what you do not want: to deteriorate.

With cancer we can feel a profound loss of meaning. The year before I was diagnosed in 2010, I had hit a milestone. I had written and published my first travel memoir, booked successful, riotously fun book launches in various cities and had done a long tour of regional signings. A film director expressed interest in adapting the book into a movie and he'd traveled a long way to develop a script with me. I had never worked with more dedication or determination for anything in my entire life; I felt both exhausted and exhilarated. This was my driving force and my true heart's calling—and an exit plan out of a lifelong career that had turned sour and stale.

When I found the cancerous lump eight months after my launch, I felt like I had been hit by a tidal wave. The news rocked me to the core of my being and all of the delicious momentum came to an abrupt halt.

What was life about anyway?

I entered a lingering 'dark night of the soul,' wondering if I had any purpose in life. I was disheartened to find myself submerged in a blue funk long after treatment and recovery.

I have heard depression defined as a devaluation of self. Unfortunately, cancer can propagate seeds of self-deprecation. It can feel like your body has let you down and you are now defective. But I remind you that cancer can bring unexpected gifts by steering you in a new direction.

Explore your feelings with someone you trust; sometimes a professional is easiest because then you do not have to be burdened over scaring a loved one. Express your fears, your tears, your anger, and also your laughter. I have driven to empty parking lots to scream and cry at the top of my lungs in the privacy of my car. I have sworn at God. Let go of any misgivings about yelling out your pain. It can offer you a much-needed release.

In her book, *The Artist's Way*, Julia Cameron touts a powerful exercise called 'The Morning Pages' for clearing blocks to creativity. What I have discovered in this process of spewing on the page is catharsis. Free-flow journaling, without censorship, is an effective way to release pent-up emotions and to clear them from your body and mind.

Cameron recommends writing at least two full pages (8 ½ x 11) first thing in the morning. On paper, there is no one to judge your thoughts and feelings, no one to placate you with platitudes and "there, there."

If you let yourself run free with anything that comes into your mind (even utter nonsense), you will become aware of things you did not even know you felt. Repetitive patterns will emerge. Some days, 'f—k cancer' may be all you feel compelled to write.

This process cleanses your mind of those inner gremlins that drag you down. Keep your journal well hidden from prying eyes so that you feel completely safe to write whatever you want and need to put on the page. The closest confidante you have is your inner spirit. I have kept a journal since Cancer II that I call *The Catalyst Chronicles*, one that is filled with my pain, my awe, my anger, and my gratitude.

Lastly, you may want to write out a happiness list and look at it often. This is everything you love and all that makes you happy.

If you need something for depression and do not want to take pharmaceutical drugs, a therapist friend of mine did extensive research on natural formulas. She discovered L-Theanine taken with 5 HTP can be as, or more, effective than antidepressants. This combination does not have the negative side effects of drugs, and it has markedly improved my mood. Note: high doses of 5 HTP can make you drowsy. If you are not sleeping well, research melatonin, and discuss these combinations with a holistic practitioner.

38

Purpose

"Man cannot stand a meaningless life."
—Carl Jung

When asked what the meaning of life is, channeler Bashar says that, at its essence, life has no inherent meaning. It is we who brand it with our own personal definition. Every experience or circumstance in our lives is something that we have assigned significance to—good or bad, happy or sad. One man's heaven is another man's hell.

A sense of purpose is essential for the will to remain on Earth with a sense of quality. It need not be grandiose. It can be a simple hobby, an athletic endeavor, growing a garden, singing, playing a musical instrument, or volunteering. Your spiritual practice or your religion may give your life meaning. Being a loving mother or grandmother who gives a family a nurturing nucleus can bring a deep contentment and has tremendous value to others. A seemingly mundane job can be infused with great purpose by setting an intention to brighten people's day while performing it.

Martin Luther King Jr. said it perfectly when he stated:

> *"... even if it falls your lot to be a street sweeper, go on out and sweep streets like Michelangelo painted pictures; sweep streets like Handel and Beethoven composed music; sweep streets like Shakespeare wrote poetry; sweep streets so well that all the hosts of heaven and earth will have to pause and say, 'Here lived a great street sweeper who swept his job well.'*
>
> *If you can't be a pine on the top of a hill*
> *Be a scrub in the valley—but be*
> *The best little scrub on the side of the rill,*
> *Be a bush if you can't be a tree.*
> *If you can't be a highway just be a trail*
> *If you can't be the sun be a star;*

It isn't by size that you win or you fail—
Be the best of whatever you are."

Purpose is not about chasing ephemeral success. It is about what profoundly moves you. It is the lifeblood of the soul's calling. When you serve others in some small way, it can satiate your spirit in a way that nothing else can. Contribution brings satisfaction.

Your life is your masterpiece—a "platform" in which you transmit that which you stand for. You may wish to create a personal mission statement that embodies who you are going forward. I have a mission statement and I have taken on a song as the theme for my life (*Vivir mi Vida*, Marc Anthony).

Do you have a bucket list? If not, start dreaming. Write things down. Even though the present moment is all that really counts, give yourself things to look forward to. Follow your excitement; whatever gives your stomach feel-good butterflies; anything that catches your eye and ignites your passion; the things that cause your heart to sing—these are the pursuits of your soul.

Sometimes your personality takes you on a goose chase far away from your innate yearnings. I learned at a young age, after my first diagnosis, that status and corporate climbing is of little importance to me. Being busy holds no value. Creative expression, however, brings tremendous meaning to my life. Small things give my life depth; spotting a rare bald eagle circling overhead on a walk; catching a full night rainbow; a heartfelt compliment from a stranger; finding a pristine white feather; sharing delectable food with a friend; attending a spontaneous event with cool people. Reacquaint yourself with all of things that give your life a rich context.

When conquering cancer is a driving purpose in your life, you can still follow your joy, and plan for the future. When you pursue the things that spark passion within, you find purpose.

Hold a precious vision of your Mecca. It can give you the patience and fortitude to see you through to the other side of suffering.

The Yellow Brick Path to Your Purpose

03/28/2014

"The purpose of life is a life of purpose."
—Robert Bryne

After attending a big writing conference in February, I decided to do an audit of my book writing efforts. I avoid numbers like I would flesh-eating disease and haven't done a proper check-in (Amazon stats) for a long while.

Most of what we are taught about business is about process, and everything I was trained for in my sales career was about logical, steadfast method. When I say process, I mean the mechanics of managing a successful business or career.

As the book industry—and the world—changes at a dizzying pace, we, as writers, are inundated with what we *must* do to succeed. Having been indoctrinated for so many years, and achieving a high level of success in sales by the A+B=C program, I have been a diligent and obedient student.

I could show you my four websites and write you a 100-page report on everything I have done, by the book, including the creation of an extensive marketing plan that became the example by which all future classes at a business school I attended use as a guideline.

So what did the audit reveal? A staggering defiance of the laws of physics. If a mathematician were to calculate my extensive efforts over the past umpteen years and determine what my results should be based on the law of averages, she/he would tell me that I have broken all laws of probability. What I discovered was that I could likely have done as well sitting under a coconut tree soliciting the odd passerby.

I have friends who are successful via a strict adherence to process. I have friends succeeding through radical non-conformity. And I have friends beating their heads against the same unyielding cement wall to live a painful and confusing reality.

Which brings me to the pursuit of our purpose. I believe everyone comes here with a unique gift, or gifts, to use and to share.

I had a life-altering AH-HA epiphany eighteen years ago while I was on a gondola in Venice. A stranger saw who I was before I knew who I was. As we floated down a dark canal, she blurted out in her deep Southern drawl, "We think you're really a famous authoress traveling incognito and you're just not telling us!"

I had been a voracious reader since childhood and realized, in that magnificent Italian moment, that I had always wanted to be a writer, but had not given myself permission to be one.

The following year I began to write and self-publish while working full-time in a sales career. *Destinations Extraordinaire* is not just a small business idea; it is what I believe to be my life's purpose, and my raison d'etre.

After reviewing my audit, I am wondering if maybe I am off base. Or … maybe I am going about it all wrong.

Do you believe you have a purpose? Do you believe you are living it? Do you care? And the big question: if you were given a month to live, do you feel you have fulfilled your life's mission?

I have always been on a quest for meaning, but since another harsh brush with my mortality, this question is the theme of my existence:

Why am I here?
Our purpose could be something less grand than we imagine. My mum has frequently stated that she has never known or fulfilled her purpose. I beg to differ—emphatically. She has been a 'Mother Hen of Excellence' and gave us a sense of balance and love in an often-tumultuous family life. She has an innate sense of goodness and generosity and has instilled many values that have served her three chickadees well. Now she has reassigned all of that good mothering to her six grandchildren who revel in a deep sense of safety and love in her care.

While doing some research on 'finding your purpose' I came across a blog post called, *How to Discover Your Purpose in About 20 Minutes*[1]. When I read the instructions, I thought the concept was an interesting one, but that I would definitely not cry, as the writer claimed I would. Because I have spent innumerable hours pondering and journaling on this topic, it was a speedy exercise. Within a minute, I was in tears. (I recommend you give it a try if you're at all interested in finding your purpose.)

---

1   http://www.stevepavlina.com/blog/2005/01/
how-to-discover-your-life-purpose-in-about-20-minutes/

For graduation night at business school, we were asked to write a letter of commitment to ourselves and recite it aloud. It is a worthy task for clarifying what is most important to you. This was mine ...

My self-commitment is to:

> *Rebuild my life through my writing and speaking. My vision is to create a business to support myself while living a completely authentic life that honors my values.*
>
> *Investigate beautiful planet Earth while inspiring, sharing insights, entertaining, revealing the soul, and promoting compassion through storytelling.*
>
> *Excellence: a commitment to ongoing learning, and to improving my writing, artistic, and speaking skills.*
>
> *Challenge the status quo and be a pioneer by incorporating play, pleasure, joy, and love into business.*
>
> *Be a goodwill ambassador as I make my way through the world.*
>
> *Continue to stretch myself by doing things that I'm afraid of, but that will grow me and inspire others to do the same.*
>
> *And lastly, to make enough money so that I don't have to do my own damn bookkeeping!*

Possibly the Universe is telling me to toss method and the myriad rules to the wind for a while. My surrender after last year's flood exposed a sweet secret. Pragmatism and process are not always the way. I learned that magical things can happen when you just relax, listen to your heart, and allow.

There sometimes comes a point when we need to do a 360. When you have proven to yourself beyond a shadow of a doubt that following convention is not bringing you to your life's mission the way you had envisioned, it might be time to play by a different set of rules. For someone who is addicted to plodding along the path of process—which means throwing a lot of poop at the wall to see what sticks—it may be a formidable challenge to shift perspective, but it is one worth testing.

Do you feel alive each day? Excited? Exhilarated? If you find that you are fighting your way against a strong current and going nowhere fast, or feel utterly uninspired, maybe it's time to turn the game upside down.

After Dorothy had tried every which way to find the road back home,

Glinda the Good Witch told her, "You've always had the power, my dear. You had it all along."

Maybe instead of strategies and tactics and dodging flying monkeys, asking for the guidance of our White Witch (divinity) and clicking our ruby slippers (our higher wisdom) with faith will spawn better results than following the herd's methodology.

More active gratitude, visualization, meditation, and heart work—less marketing. More listening for the guidance—less busy work. For others it may be letting go of doing the same things over and over while seeking different results (the definition of insanity, according to Einstein).

The pot of gold at the end of the Yellow Brick Road, for me, is life with a deep sense of purpose, peace, play, and joy. How I get there or where I land may, after all, be none of my business.

The Yellow Brick Path to Your Purpose
http://wp.me/p2ACw4-ma
lifebyheart.wandasthilaire.com

39

Movement, Music, and the Breath

"Beethoven tells you what it's like to be Beethoven and Mozart tells you what it's like to be human. Bach tells you what it's like to be the Universe."
—Douglas Adams

I've heard that sitting is the new smoking. Our bodies were not designed to be sedentary and remain seated in office chairs or cars all day. Our lymphatic systems need movement to circulate and cleanse toxins and free radicals from our systems. When we sit for too long, we shallow breathe and the body requires an abundance of oxygen for wellbeing.

Even though you may be struggling with pain, moving your body will help your immune system and speed recovery. What you are able to do will vary from person to person based on your condition. But do not let the illness halt your movement completely. You could end up with other complications if you lie or sit for extended periods.

Many cancer centers offer gentle yoga specifically designed for cancer patients. You can walk slowly in a park or along a river or lakeshore. If you are at home, put on your favorite music and gently sway or dance. Dancing can help release trapped emotions. Blending movement with stirring music is something that helps remind you life is worth living.

Cancer can steal your essence. Music reconnects you with who you are and where you come from. It hits you deep in the heart. It can excite or move you to the core of your being. Music can be better than any chemical sedative to comfort and soothe you. It is also a powerful form of therapy that promotes wellness.

And it's as close as a click of the mouse: YouTube houses pre-made playlists for almost any genre, era, or mood. Relaxation and meditative music will calm you when you are worried. Classical music can stimulate creativity and naturally quiet the monkey mind. You may want to listen to the music from your youth or a playful period of your life that brings back good memories. I have created a playlist of '90s dance music for when I want an energy boost. It takes me back to carefree days and crazy nights.

Get concert DVDs of your favorite singers or groups and watch them over dinner. If, for example, you like contemporary classical, you can find live concert recordings of Il Divo, Il Volo, The Tenors, Andrea Bocelli, Sarah Brightman, Katherine Jenkins, Alfio, Ólafur Arnalds, and Josh Groban.

If you like to sing, go for a drive and put on some of your favorite sing-along-songs. I like to go to the mountains and belt out tunes all the way. If you play an instrument, now is a good time to be the star in your own private performances. Song writing at this time can be an outlet for expressing emotions that are hard to deal with. Some of the world's best songs were written during tumultuous times.

Have your favorite playlists on hand at the hospital or treatment center to help with anxiety. Use hypnosis or meditative music to fall asleep if you suffer from insomnia.

I used to think breathing classes and techniques were an unnecessary waste of time. We all have to breathe in order to live, so what's the big deal? What I have come to realize is that I am a shallow breather and under stress, my breathing becomes constricted, as is the case for many of us. The body loves oxygen and it is only because of our sedentary and stressful lifestyles that we need to relearn how to breathe. Proper breathing exercises can also dislodge stuck emotions. I was surprised to see a weight loss book with breathing techniques as the method (*Jumpstart Your Metabolism: How To Lose Weight By Changing The Way You Breathe*, Pam Grout). She has listed some effective breathing exercises that promote good health.

The use of breathing techniques while in nature is a relaxing way to rejuvenate—cancer does not like an oxygen rich environment. Dr. Otto Warburg, President, Institute of Cell Physiology, and Nobel Prize Winner states: *"Deep breathing techniques which increase oxygen to the cell are the most important factors in living a disease free and energetic life. Remember: where cells get enough oxygen, cancer will not, cannot occur."*

This link to a stirring documentary explores the powerful effects of music, and follows social worker Dan Cohen, as he fights against a broken healthcare system. In this film you will discover the miraculous effects of music on humans. Alive Inside: www.aliveinside.us

I promise you this gorgeous song will comfort you in your darkest hours: 100,000 Angels by Bliss:
https://youtu.be/VhfMgVonRjk

This loop of Beethoven's Symphony No. 7, 2nd movement is said to have healing effects on the body and mind:
https://youtu.be/9AjFN4uD3h4

The Sweet, Sweet Sound of Music
10/31/2013

"Without music, life would be a mistake."
—Friedrich Nietzche

I come from a musical household. When I was young, there would be mornings we were awakened by the sound of a strumming guitar, a stomping foot, and my dad singing a Johnny Cash or Elvis tune.

My dad played in bands and my parents, married young, were party-goers and party-throwers when I was small. At family get-togethers, my uncle Mel and my dad would sing and play guitars into the wee hours of the morning. Dad also had a banjo, a ukulele, and a violin.

My little sister would dance at parties and get "tips" because she was so frigging cute while I would sit steaming in a corner—coveting the cash and her pluck—because I was too inhibited to follow suit.

My mum would always hum or sing while she did chores around the house, and my sister, much to my consternation, would belt out ditties operatically in the bathtub when we were in our teens. Incidentally, my mum's long-time partner still isn't used to my sister, mum, and I breaking into tune when some subject reminds us of a particular song.

At twelve, I wanted to learn the piano, but we got a small organ instead and my parents hired a bald, wheezing, fat man with extreme halitosis to teach me. He sat next to me on the piano bench; that didn't last long.

My brother did learn the organ, but we never heard a peep out of him and only recently discovered that the kid has some awesome singing pipes.

There was a lot of fighting between my parents and it very well could have been the joyful respite of music that kept us all from going Looney Tunes.

Once I got over myself, I loved to sing. Fortunately the friends I had in my twenties liked to do the same. We would karaoke often and when we were all married and living in nice homes, we would throw weekend parties and set up a "lounge." I was gifted a karaoke machine and microphones for my thirtieth birthday—the ultimate present for a fledgling songbird.

Typically the guys would play pool or darts and we girls would sing our hearts out. Sometimes we'd even get ovations from the boys for an extra good rendition of Reba McEntire or Patsy Cline.

I remember when I had invited a good friend from work to a party, and extended the invitation to her new husband. He was mortified by our singing and left early. We didn't care. We *loved* to sing and spent hours at it. It was powerful play for the soul.

I have a useless talent for remembering lyrics and can likely sing you 1000 songs correctly. I think I developed it from entertaining myself on excessively long road trips over a lifetime in sales.

I even walked down the aisle on my wedding day to *"The Power of Love"*[1] (a la 1984 Jennifer Rush rendition), which I had secretly recorded for my husband. On long trips he would ask me to sing to him and I would happily oblige.

I asked my dad to sing at my wedding, but he was nervous about being too emotional to do it well, so opted out. Instead of clinking glasses, anyone who wanted to see a bridal kiss at the reception had to sing a song. My friends embraced the concept and people got up in droves to perform. My dad, realizing there was nothing to fear in that crowd, surprised us all with a remarkable a cappella version of *The Hawaiian Wedding Song*[2]. I don't think there was a dry eye in the house.

I started singing one day on a road trip with a new boyfriend, après divorce, and he nearly jumped out of his seat. His father was a well-known doctor and their childhood home had been a stodgy, academic environment where nobody *ever* broke out into tune.

When I moved to Calgary, the music in me, in a manner of speaking, died. I arrived after a massive heartbreak and became mute. I stopped singing in the car or shower. My voice became thin and weak from emotional trauma. My new friends thought I was somewhat crazed when I finally felt a stirring and suggested a karaoke night. Without song mates, the joy and playfulness of singing came to an end.

I have had blissful periods of intense dancing because the music

---

1 https://youtu.be/5boRQcTvnwU
2 https://youtu.be/Vljvem9AJII

moved me. When I was sixteen and seventeen, I loved to dance (illegally) at cabarets to the disco hits of the day—*Dancing Queen, Carwash, The Hustle, Disco Inferno, Brick House* …

When I turned eighteen, I started going to country bars and became a dancing cowgirl—my friends and I were the first in Edmonton to learn the 'Cotton-Eyed-Joe' and we spent at least three nights a week two-stepping our butts off with the urban cowboys of the day.

One year, at a luxurious weeklong sales meeting that was held in New Orleans, our team got to enjoy the best of Cajun everything. I had never heard live zydeco music[1] before and I stayed out all seven nights just to dance. I had blisters and almost couldn't walk by the last day. I ate my way through N'awlins eating rich Creole food, yet lost three pounds.

In my thirties, I discovered Latin music and that stuck. When you get a taste of Cuba, the sensual beat and soul of *son cubano* gets under your skin and won't go away.

And, of course, music is the master of seduction, the language of love.

One night in Mexico, a group of us were at an outdoor restaurant where a band played traditional Peruvian music. The talented lead singer was a beautiful, indigenous Mexican. He looked like a regal Apache in a movie who'd just dismounted a stallion. Much to my girlfriend Gina's amusement, he and I could not stop staring at each other. We went for a drink that night and on my subsequent trips there, he would sing traditional Spanish songs to me and I would melt like liquid butter. I was besotted.

When a couple I know from Edmonton asked me if I would be interested in a date weekend with a tall, stunning Italian opera singer from NYC who was in town to perform at the Winspear Theatre, which included an invitation to the after party, I was in the car headed there faster than you can say *Ciao, Baby*.

A simple song can bring people together. One day while writing in a café, I heard a phenomenal piano piece. A couple sat next to me working on their Macs, he a dapper dude in a bowler, she an Eastern European beauty. The song reminded me of a haunting song I had heard in Venice on a rainy night and it captivated me. I asked who the composer was. I was thrilled to discover that the piece was his! I ordered a CD, we met for coffee for the delivery, and it was platonic love at first sight. Had it

---

1   https://youtu.be/MH2eRRh4Bls

not been for a song, I would not know Francis and Sanja, a very rich addition to my life.

A song can make you weep, evoke a flash of memories, cause your heart to flutter, send shivers down your spine, or move you to the core. It can inspire you and it can heal you. A song can become your "anthem" for a particular period of your life and can narrate your story. It can pump you up or make you smile on a dreary day. It can also irritate the hell out of you if it breaks your equilibrium.

Even if you do not understand the lyrics, a foreign song can transcend language; you just *know* what the song is about because you feel it. A song can unexpectedly become a worldwide phenomenon because it strikes a universal chord.

Music is the soul of the world. If you have placed it as a background noise in your life, bring it into the forefront. Seek new music. Be open to introductions of what others are listening to. Listen for something that moves you. Find something you cannot sit still to and dance, dance, dance. Let loose with a good song in the shower—sing at the top of your lungs in the car—the extra oxygen alone will make your body hum. It's natural medicine.

I know when my spirit is buoyed because I begin to sing again. A life without music that moves you is black and white. Be sure to color your world with the sweet, sweet sound of music.

The Sweet, Sweet Sound of Music
http://wp.me/p2ACw4-iF
lifebyheart.wandasthilaire.com

40

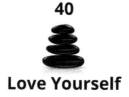

Love Yourself

"As you love yourself, life loves you back. I don't think it has a choice either. I can't explain how it works, but I know it to be true."
—Kamal Ravikant[1]
Love Yourself Like Your Life Depends On It[2]

The love of self is a topic of colossal magnitude. Entire volumes have been dedicated to its crucial role in our personal growth, our health, and our level of contentment. When we attain true self-love, it transmutes the quality of life in unimaginable ways.

As trite as it may sound, Whitney Houston's song, *"the greatest love of all's inside of me"* is a profound truth: you need not seek love from outside of yourself. Before self-love comes self-acceptance. You choose your thoughts and feelings about yourself, and illness can be a new path to self-love if you have veered off course. It can be *the* most important internal shift for your healing.

If you want an optimally happy and healthy life, you need to be your own biggest cheerleader. When you fall in love with someone, there is a magical chemical that pulses through your body called oxytocin. When you show yourself compassion; when you "fall in love" with yourself, you manufacture that same life-affirming drug.

Louise Hay, the mother of affirmations, discovered in her coaching forty-some years ago that self-love is the linchpin in solving almost any issue. She recommends mirror work as a foundational practice. It is such a simple technique that it seems almost too silly to consider. But it is powerful. It can be uncomfortable at first, but look into your own eyes and say, *I love you. <Your name> I really love you. I accept you. I approve of you.*

In Louise Hay's movie, *You Can Heal Your Life,* one woman shared how she had spent three months doing mirror work along with daily mega

1   https://www.goodreads.com/author/show/6422677.Kamal_Ravikant
2   https://www.goodreads.com/work/quotes/21367410

affirmations and was healed of breast cancer. She admitted to being harshly critical of herself and found this practice transformational.

Self-love has been a challenge on my life's path. I have berated myself for many perceived failures, flops, and fiascos. But 'failure' is only a perspective—one that can be changed. Self-forgiveness, self-love, and self-compassion are critical, and I am learning to look at my missteps from a different angle. I understand that we are each a work in progress, moment-by-moment, doing the best we can with the knowledge that we have at the time.

As I mentioned earlier, comparing yourself to others is a swift and sure path to misery and it caustically erodes self-love—trust me, I know. We can feel like a princess or king in a tiny apartment just as easily as we can in a grandiose castle. We can be stunningly attractive with an extra 20 pounds if we believe ourselves to be so. Keep your eyes on your own journey and not that of another.

Own all aspects of yourself. Learn to accept your imperfections. Love yourself in all of your pain, your mistakes, and your weaknesses. See your beauty and your goodness and give yourself blazing credit for all of your successes, big and small. Spend an afternoon celebrating you. Write a list of all of your accomplishments, your amazing character traits, and your talents. Do you have a wicked sense of humor? Cook a scrumptious paella? Are you a party planner extraordinaire? Or are you the fly fisherman of the century? Focus on this list when you need a lift and dump perceived flaws into the trash file.

There is a simple Hawaiian prayer based on something called Ho'oponopono. It is considered to be a method of stress reduction and is extremely potent in healing. The prayer is directed toward the self.

Thank you
Please forgive me
I'm sorry
I love you
Repeat often.

Almost everything in the world tells you that you are not enough, just as you are. I write these pages not to tell you that you need to change the fundamental you; I write to remind you that once you exhume the layers of expectations, and self-judgments, and feelings of wrongness—all the years of crud that have lead you to believe you're not good enough or are too broken—that you are so very lovable, so incredibly deserving. Once the debris is unearthed and cleared away, what lies underneath the excavation is a specular city of splendor—*you*.

When you embrace divinity's reality, you cannot help but love yourself because you know that you are an intrinsic part of everything. It is erroneous to think that you and you alone are unloved or unlovable. Hold yourself in reverence and love yourself the way you would a precious newborn child.

If everything in the Universe is love and is loved—down to a tiny, iridescent hummingbird—*then why not you?*

How Do I Love Thee?
10/18/2012

"You yourself, as much as anybody in the entire Universe, deserve your love and affection."
—Buddha

My sister recently told me about a conversation she'd had with my 14-year-old nephew. In the height of pubescent angst, he bemoaned being average; he wasn't smart enough, good looking enough, and did not meet his own expectations at sports.

Although the kid, when wearing his hair Bieber-esque, is often told he looks exactly like the teen idol; took it upon himself to study the animal kingdom encyclopedia when he was 9 years of age and then moved on to the entire history of the world and can tell you about any species or era; and recently won MVP at a hockey tournament, his mother asked him, "Can't you accept being average at some things?"

"No! Mediocrity is a guy with a bunch of losers behind him and a bunch of assholes ahead of him!"

"So you want to join the ranks of the assholes?"

"Yes!"

It begins young, our feelings of being not enough. Here is an exceptional kid who considers himself extremely ordinary.

This summer, as I was gathering my bags to take into my apartment, I witnessed a loud domestic dispute on the street. At first, my concern was that the woman might be in danger. I hovered around my car to ensure there was no physical violence. Imagine my shock when I saw the women actually punch *herself* in the face three times. Hard. The man left in dismay, her trailing behind begging him not to leave. It was obvious, and deeply disturbing, that this woman was suffering from acute self-loathing.

When the Dalai Lama was asked—while speaking in India with a group of Western philosophers, psychologists, and scientists—what his thoughts were about self-hatred, he asked the interpreter to repeat the question because he could not grasp the concept. At the end of the session he said, "I thought I had a very good acquaintance with the mind, but now I feel quite ignorant. I find this very, very strange."

On the sometimes-rocky 'life by heart' path, self-love and acceptance becomes an integral part of the journey. Without it, doubt, fear, and confusion override contentment and happiness.

So why is self-love sometimes so elusive? Aside from the obvious—the onslaught of images and stories of perfection and wealth by the media and advertisers—here are a few thoughts about what can tarnish our self-image.

Our marriage or relationship is as much fun as a chapped bum. Not having the courage to move on from a destructive or dysfunctional relationship can cause a loss of self-respect.

We are single and we appear to have a cloak of invisibility around the opposite sex. It can be mighty hard to muster up feeling like a god/goddess when you are being overlooked, and it can create self-doubt about your attraction factor.

Every pair of jeans we own have become 'camel toe central.' If exercise is a bad word and we are pushing the envelope on our healthy weight limits, we can feel like we are failing ourselves, and physical lethargy can affect our emotions.

We are prone to comparing ourselves to others who appear to be in a much better position than we are. We know we are not supposed to compare ourselves to others, but when we fall into the trap of envy, it can erode our self-confidence.

We are harboring a dark secret. This one isn't me; I am a memoirist who can't keep a secret about my life if I tried. If the secret is about you, it's in the vault. If it's about me—no way, José. Shame around secrets can hugely affect our feelings toward ourselves. Volumes have been written about shame around secrets and their destructive effects.

We feel like we've been rotating on a fence post for far too long. Being stuck in any area of life can leave a person feeling ineffective and essentially disempowered. Feeling powerless can have a significant impact on self-love.

We need a shovel to get through our clutter. A messy home or office can wreak havoc with our moods and can sometimes offer us a chaotic glimpse of what's going on in our minds.

We are living a lie. Whether it is a job we loathe or some aspect of ourselves we have shelved and hidden for fear of disapproval, a voice will most certainly nag at us to be true to ourselves, no matter what others may think.

We are up to our eyeballs in procrastination. A heap of projects left unfinished or "to dos" that really need to be done can leave us with a constant residue of discomfort and self-criticism.

We are so broke we can't even afford to pay attention. If a major focus in our lives is how we are going to cover our basic needs or we have a big debt load, our self-esteem can plummet.

Some of these conditions can be overwhelming, so much so that we become immobilized. I have been a student of self-help, metaphysics, and philosophy for years and what I have gleaned is that at this juncture, instead of trying to tackle the seemingly insurmountable, bump up the self-love.

Over the course of her long career, Louise Hay has helped millions of people find their way out of poverty, illness, and problematic relationships. She maintains that the root cause of all problems is a lack of self-love. Her simple prescription: healing your life through affirmations.

Are affirmations corny and trite or do they work? Can you "fake it 'til you make it?" It has been scientifically proven that how we feel affects the rhythms of our hearts and can be recorded at a long distance from our bodies[1]. We are emitting messages and feelings to the world at all times. If our message shifts to one of self-compassion, will life's challenges morph? Quite likely, I have discovered.

Appreciation is another concept that comes up in many teachings— looking at ourselves as "enough" and at our lives from a place of sufficiency and gratitude rather than deficiency and dissatisfaction. Oprah swears by writing a list of everything you are thankful for at day's end and categorically states that this one thing alone can change your life in surprising ways.

If you are up for bedtime gratitude journaling, be sure to include *you*—the things that are awesome about you: your achievements, your kindnesses, your body, your character, the life you have created, your mind, your resourcefulness.

As always, what the world needs now is love sweet love. And it all begins within.

---

1   The Heartmath Solution/Doc Childre and Howard Martin

How Do I Love Thee
http://wp.me/p2ACw4-aI
lifebyheart.wandasthilaire.com

41

Vulnerability

"Vulnerability is our most accurate measurement of courage."
—Brené Brown

I view vulnerability as the state of allowing yourself to be seen and heard in your full truth—in your strengths and your weaknesses. I also see it as the willingness to love deeply, without borders or constraints. When you are vulnerable, you give others the opportunity to exhale a huge metaphorical sigh; as you bare your soul, another is given the freedom to let down any façades and bare theirs.

Cancer is something that either cracks you open or curls you into contraction. Vulnerability is not comfortable, but it is a profound human experience that can bring a tremendous richness and depth to life in the midst of your tsunami.

I am not suggesting that you shout your circumstances and feelings from the highest rooftop. We must take great care with whom we share our vulnerability: our deepest pain, and our darkest story. As researcher and author Brené Brown advises, some people do not deserve our vulnerability because they do not know how to honor it. You know who those people are in your life. But there are others who love you and are cheering for your victory. These are the people with whom you can open your heart.

When a friend sent out an email requesting financial assistance for me during cancer two, I was initially mortified that I'd agreed to it. I am a strong, independent woman who has been single for most of my life. I felt ashamed that I was in a position to require help. I was worried that people would think less of me or assume I was frittering away their contributions on nonsense. It was also painful because a few of my closest friends did not partake, while perfect strangers did. I allowed myself to be more vulnerable than I had ever been in my life. I asked for what I needed in other ways. I did not always get it, but I had the courage to ask.

Many years ago I attended a personal development workshop with 35 other participants. On the second day we were given an exercise that required us to mill around the room and give feedback to every attendee about our first impressions of them. We had to be completely honest and we could not avoid anyone. A whopping 90% of the feedback I received was that I was intimidating. Men especially expressed the sentiment that my demeanor was threatening. A young man in the class (still a teen) who had just lost his mother said I scared the daylights out of him. I was stunned. I am an ultra-sensitive person and care deeply about people. I consider myself marshmallow soft.

Over the course of the workshop, all of our defenses were decimated. We laughed, we cried, we enacted skits contrary to our personality, we had to be silly—we were stretched far out of our comfort zones and our true selves were exposed—raw and naked. By day five of the workshop I realized that I had developed a powerful suit of armor that I lived behind (and still do at times). As I dropped my "weapons" the men's response to me turned around completely.

The most poignant moment of that experience came after the graduation dinner. Our group was still high from the experience so we decided to gather at someone's house to celebrate. I snuggled into a huge circular wicker chair and much to my amazement, the young man who had been terrified of me came over and curled up in my arms—and *fell asleep*. He was struggling with the death of his mum and he chose me as a safe place to let go. I was honored and moved to tears. Because I was forced to abandon my mask and be myself in all of my weakness, my bad, my beauty, and my good, I became the haven instead of the landmine.

Vulnerability is, contrary to what we fear, an attractor. The times that I have allowed myself to be wholly vulnerable are the moments I have experienced the most love, the biggest joy, and a palpable expansion of gratitude in my heart. Our vulnerability is what allows our inner magnificence to shine through.

When you drop your defensiveness and the fortress you have placed around yourself, you can breathe. Really breathe. A tightness that you did not even know you held is released. Cancer is an opportunity to get as real as you have ever been. People can only truly know you, understand you, and connect with you on a deep heart level when you show up as yourself. Dissolving walls and removing the shell that you have developed over a lifetime can liberate you.

TEDxHouston | The Power of Vulnerability
Brené Brown
https://youtu.be/iCvmsMzlF7o

The Upside of Vulnerability
04/19/2013

If the shell of a heart hardens to the unfairness and injustices dealt it,
does it sever the lifeline that nourishes the beauty and tenderness that live inside?
To carry a jaded and cynical heart seems a most heavy and sad burden.
May we survive these trials only to become more resilient
yet still full of love and buoyancy.
—Wanda St. Hilaire
Of Love, Life and Journeys

vul·ner·a·ble (vlnr—bl)
a*dj.*
1.
a. Susceptible to physical or emotional injury.
b. Susceptible to attack.
c. Open to censure or criticism; assailable.

Quite a number of posts back, I was about to write about vulnerability when I was put to the challenge to be more transparent and open in my writing by both my school coach and mentor and so instead, I took the gauntlet and wrote with even greater vulnerability.

Upon my last post (*Premeditated Acts of Kindness and Purpose Driven Beauty*[1]), my mum wrote me and in her protective, good-mothering nature, suggested that maybe I should reveal less about my life and circumstances. Especially in light of the fact that I would like to find love once again, she expressed concern that my raw honesty might scare off any would-be suitor should he read the blog.

And therein lies the splendid paradox of vulnerability.

One of the reasons why many people who want to write do not do so is because of the potential rejection, ridicule, and criticism. Publishing my writing for the world to see is one of the most vulnerable acts I have ever committed. When I wrote poetry in the midst of the most

---

1 http://lifebyheart.wandasthilaire.com/gallery/
premeditated-acts-of-kindness-and-purpose-driven-beauty/

intense heartbreak of my life, I never dreamed I would share it. But as fate would have it, I did.

By no stretch of the imagination is it Keats[1] or Shelley[2], but in sharing it, I allowed women who read it to own their concealed anguish and realize they were not alone. The men who read it were visibly moved and felt a greater understanding of women and of how their own actions may have contributed to more fallout than they had considered.

In being open to the risk of criticism by publishing it, *Of Love, Life and Journeys* became a bestseller (by Canadian poetry standards) and hit the 'Top Twenty Books of 2004' (#10) at McNally Robinson Books, which gave me a great sense of accomplishment.

Writing a travel memoir[3] that was romantic in nature, something I had wanted to do for a long time, required digging into a profound well of vulnerability. To put myself out there—naked for all to see my biases, blemishes, and behavior—took a tremendous amount of courage.

But again, in doing so, I have received numerous emails from women and men telling me that *The Cuban Chronicles* had been a catalyst for their own AH-HA epiphanies or how much they appreciated the honesty and frankness with which I wrote it and that they too felt the many emotions with me along the journey. This feedback brings me bursts of bliss and keeps me believing.

The fear of disapproval can put a halt to many potentially great adventures, projects, or pursuits. I have tossed aside my need for knowing the outcome and for all manner of security to do what I value most—write—for whom I value most: real and good people. My tallest challenge is to live with the mystery in trust.

A quote by Anaïs Nin resonates loudest with my quest: "And the day came when the risk to remain tight in a bud was more painful than the risk it took to blossom."

Brené Brown, a PhD researcher who has spent a decade studying vulnerability, courage, worthiness, and shame, says that vulnerability is the birthplace of everything—of innovation, creativity, and change. Think about it. Your grandest moments were likely born from your bravest vulnerability. Mine were.

In a highly unexpected twist, Brown's Ted Talk, *The Power of*

1 http://en.wikipedia.org/wiki/John_Keats
2 http://en.wikipedia.org/wiki/Percy_Bysshe_Shelley
3 http://writewaycafe.com/the-cuban-chronicles/

Vulnerability[1], went viral. In it she shares a deeply personal story about where her studies and statistics took her on her own journey. I speculate that the reason the talk has had 6 million hits (to date) is that we are all seeking the same relief from our hidden fears that make us feel weak or powerless.

Anyone who has ever been seriously ill, critically injured, or been given a dire diagnosis will tell you they have experienced gaping, raw vulnerability. False pretenses fall away when we are faced with intense physical pain or our mortality. But our greatest gifts come in these somber hours when we learn how strong we really are, the depth of our faith, and what we truly value.

Not wanting to appear weak or be susceptible to hurt, it is in romance that many of us put on our heaviest suit of armor to hide any flaws or frailties. Yet the only way to intimacy and whole-hearted relationships is through being emotionally exposed, without guarantees or certainty.

Adele sang about the agony of love in *Someone Like You*. The incredible vulnerability in her song writing caused her album, *21*, to surpass Michael Jackson's landmark *Thriller* because millions of us could relate.

Friendships and romantic liaisons remain shallow when we hide who we really are. There is no depth to a relationship when we only scratch the surface and pretend that everything is what it is not. Like eating a donut, I leave hungry and wanting for more when I visit with a friend and get only the superficial goods. I feel like I have been deprived of the honor of really knowing that person. I cannot help another if I do not know their pain or their strife. I cannot celebrate their greatness if they do not share all of themselves with me.

I watched a movie with a friend this weekend called *Hope Springs*[2], starring Tommy Lee Jones and the endlessly talented Meryl Streep. It had been labeled a comedy/drama, but my friend was in tears for a lot of the 100 minutes. It touched a sensitive nerve about her own failed marriage.

The movie epitomized the damage done to relationships and self-esteem caused by the fortresses of emotional impenetrability we build through pride and misunderstanding. Thankfully, it also revealed what lies on the other side of letting go.

I was brought up to believe that one does not air their dirty laundry

1 http://www.ted.com/talks/brene_brown_on_vulnerability.html
2 https://youtu.be/pfK8DF0AdRw

in public. It was a value my parents were brought up with and likely one that was passed down throughout the generations. However, our façades and dirty little secrets are our captors. Silence and secrecy grow like a dangerous fungus, suffocating happiness. Shame of who we are, what has happened to us, or what we have done can only be healed in light, not hidden in a dank basement of darkness.

The great cosmic joke of vulnerability is that the weaknesses we are all trying to conceal from each other, we all have. What a kicker! The paradox is that in trying to protect ourselves from hurt, we foster internal suffering. Being vulnerable means being susceptible to emotional injury, but also to astounding joy.

Rather than numb (with food, alcohol, drugs, sex, TV, shopping, or gambling) and hide our shortcomings and letdowns, we run the highest chance of finding happiness, surprises, and love in unexpected places from unexpected people when we show up and allow ourselves to be seen in our entirety.

There is emancipation in honesty. If someone does not like you or accept you based on your truth, they do not belong in your life anyway. For me, in writing with vulnerability and candor, I am allowing my life to heal and hopefully inspiring a few others along the way to do the same. For you, it may be telling your husband how you feel about your sex life. It might lie in finally dropping the mask with a good friend and speaking your shame. It could be a letting go of a need for perfection and being beyond reproach.

We all long for a sense of connection and belonging, of being seen and cherished for who we imperfectly are. What a wonderful world it would be if we all became each other's liberators by openly living life by heart and telling our story as it is, not as we think it should be.

The Upside of Vulnerability
http://wp.me/s2ACw4-957
lifebyheart.wandasthilaire.com

All the Way Down
the Rabbit Hole

42

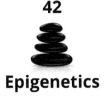

Epigenetics

"The moment you change your perception is the moment you rewrite the chemistry of your body."
—Dr. Bruce Lipton

We have been taught a model of genetic determinism—that our DNA determines our fate. Many people *expect* to get the diseases of their parents and simply await the verdict with resignation.

It has now been proven that our DNA is not on an automatic default position in our bodies. The gene's tipping point can be set off by how we live our lives: by environmental toxins, stress, addictions, poor nutrition, perpetual negative self-talk and chronic emotional rollercoasters, unhealthy lifestyles and destructive behavior, a lack of support, and trauma. These interferences mess up the function of the "housekeepers" within the body so that they are unable to repair damaged genes. Our choices matter beyond what we wish to imagine.

We may have the cancer gene, but genetic expression is something that is switched off or on—which is good news. It means we have a level of control in downregulating the gene and we are not the victims of our DNA. A woman with the breast cancer gene BRCA2 will not unequivocally get breast cancer. And women who do not have the gene, get it. We have reviewed a multitude of things that can be done to heal and to prevent a cancer recurrence and also discovered what activates a faulty gene. Instead of cutting off an entire breast, a woman can make appropriate lifestyle changes.

To further understand how genetic expression is affected by stress and lifestyle, we can delve into the world of telomeres and telomerase. Sound boring? Not really. The length and state of your telomeres are the best predictors longevity, health, and whether we look youthful or haggard.

Telomeres are the ends of chromosomes, which carry genetic information. They are like the little plastic cap on the end of shoelaces and they protect the chromosome from fraying and shortening. They deteriorate and can be damaged, which in turn causes the cells to malfunction and send the wrong signals—cues that create chronic disease and illness. Dr. Elizabeth Blackburn won the Nobel Prize in 2009 for her discovery of telomerase, the enzyme that replenishes telomeres. She states that exercise, good nutrition, healthy lifestyle, and the reduction of chronic stress helps lessen oxidative stress and helps the telomeres stay strong and long. Telomerase is activated in the presence of gratitude and self-love. Remember, your telomeres are listening.

We can literally change the composition of our blood with our perceptions on life. A long time ago after a devastating heartbreak, I returned to Canada to begin my life over again. I went for blood analysis for a small health problem. The nurse showed me the fascinating video of my live analysis and explained the various things going on in my blood. She asked me if I had recently experienced a significant emotional trauma. I was surprised by the question considering we were looking at my *blood*.

"Yes, why?" I asked.

She pointed to the images. "These cells are curled, as though they've been assaulted. It's a sign of emotional trauma."

I knew right then that we cannot escape bodily harm when we allow our emotional lives to run wild and unchecked. As Dr. Caroline Myss aptly puts it, "your biography becomes your biology."

It may be a hard pill to swallow, but your thoughts, beliefs, and emotional states can flip the switch on the genes of cancer. Your level of optimism or negativity affects your genetic expression. This is not about self-blame or guilt; it is about empowerment and accountability. Of all of the things I have previously discussed in this book, I think that the discoveries in epigenetics is one of the most exciting, because our destiny is not, as we have been lead to believe, inevitable. Our behavior and beliefs are the most significant influencer of our inner physiology.

This is why it is vital that you address whatever imbalances exist in your life. When you openly face what has led to the mis-expression of your genes, you have the opportunity to remedy the situation. The doctors will not give you a prescription for making lifestyle changes in regard to things they know nothing about, or for rectifying relationship and job issues. You know in the core of your inner world that which is not harmonious and beneficial to you.

I shared a glimpse of my cancer story in the chapter on stress. Although there is no way to prove it, I suspect that after a twenty-year triumph over the disease, it was my perceptions on circumstances and a choice to let my negative emotions overtake me that activated an already existing predisposition to cancer (breast cancer runs fatally on my father's side). I'd been hit by what felt like an assault to my self-worth in my career and prior to that, it seemed like I had attracted the lowest denominator for a romantic partner.

Those two events happened two months apart and my overall state was one of hopelessness. Less than six months later, I had a tumor in my other breast in a mirror image location of the first cancer; I'd had a clean mammogram less than two years prior and was a regular self-examiner. I share this as a cautionary tale—an unbalanced inner life *will* catch up to you. You cannot afford to put off that which you know you need to do now.

We all know someone who eats nutritiously, exercises frequently, and seems to live well, yet has been diagnosed with a disease or has had a heart attack. We are mystified. But people wear veneers that hide what goes on inside. They do not share their deep-seated resentments, their self-loathing, or their incessant cycles of discontentment. This is the secret of what most profoundly destroys our health.

We hold the power with our genetics, no matter the hand we have been dealt. We can objectively look at our lives and make new decisions that will keep imperfect genes in a state of stability.

If you want to understand the science behind epigentics, read Dr. Bruce Lipton's two books, *The Biology of Belief* and *The Honeymoon Effect*. Deepak Chopra and Rudolph Tanzi have a new book out called *Super Genes* (2016) explaining what shapes your gene activity, and Dawson Church, PhD, has written the book *The Genie in our Genes*.

Dr. Bruce Lipton YouTube
https://www.youtube.com/user/biologyofbelief

NOVA Epigentics
(Fascinating and a mention of new cutting-edge epigenetic therapy in the world of cancer.)
https://youtu.be/avWwfuJYnnI

43

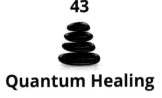

Quantum Healing

"We should never wait for science to give us permission to do the uncommon;
if we do, then we are turning science into another religion."
—Dr. Joe Dispenza

The world of science is becoming über exciting with myriad discoveries of how powerful the mind is in healing the body. In the area of neuroscience, we now know that the brain has plasticity—meaning it can change—and can be rewired at any age. It has been proven that we have the ability to form new mental habits that will heal our bodies and our lives.

Many years ago, my hero, Dr. Joe Dispenza, was a young and active chiropractor. During a triathlon in California he was flagged ahead in the biking segment of the race by a police officer. Seconds later, a Bronco traveling at 55 miles/hour hit him and dragged him down the road. He soon discovered that he had six broken vertebrae.

Dr. Joe sought various opinions from specialists about what type of surgery was required. With the possibility of a lifetime of pain and debilitation and a likely disability—and in spite of the probable chance of paralysis—he opted against all recommendations and made a radical decision to self-heal. He believed in a conscious intelligence with the power to lead him to wholeness.

Face down, he spent hours rehearsing and visualizing the rebuilding of his spine and picturing himself healed, happy, and living his active and busy life once again. He gave his body a template of healing and surrendered himself to a higher power. It was an arduous process that required incredible focus and dedication.

Naturally, doubts crept in to taunt him. But he was vigilant in paying attention to his thoughts—and of who he was being and how he was speaking about and reacting to his condition. If he wandered off with thoughts about all of the things that could go wrong and all of the scenarios he feared, he would begin the process all over again from the beginning.

Unbelievably, only 9 ½ weeks after he was told he might never walk again, he did get up and walk. He added a regime of energy healing, diet, and physical rehabilitation and has been active and healthy since—he even rides horses. He later understood that he had been offering the quantum field a host of optimistic future potentials and was imprinting his body with the emotional signature of health and joy. He learned that our thoughts and emotions are intrinsically linked to our destiny.

He made a promise to a higher power while healing that if walked again, he would dedicate his life to examining the mind-body connection. I have studied his books, listened to countless interviews, I attend his monthly teleclasses, and have been to one of his mind-altering progressive workshops. He is my Superman because of his tireless work around the globe to help people break free from their limiting habits and beliefs so that they heal from addictions, heartbreak, financial devastation, and illness. He shows us the *how* of quantum healing, and he does it in a highly self-empowering, non-guru-like manner that is both scientific and comprehensible.

Because of our indoctrination of the medical model that tells us healing comes from outside of ourselves, it is a stretch to wrap our minds around the idea that we can heal both small ailments and monumental diseases with the power of the mind in union with "the field." We have had the wisdom beaten out of us that we own bodies with magnificent self-healing capacity.

You have watched how your own body naturally heals a deep cut; this is just a fraction of what it is capable of with its potent ability to fight invading infections and disease. The human body is a marvel of adaptability and healing. When you add the power of the mind in conjunction with consciousness, you are limitless.

Joe Dispenza, Gregg Braden, Deepak Chopra, Bruce Lipton, Dawson Church, and many others in the field of neuroscience teach us how to become our own physicians.

Did you know that when clinical trials are done on a new drug, they are given to a control group and a placebo (an inert pill) is always given to a second group to test its effectiveness? When Dr. David Hamilton completed his PhD, he worked in the pharmaceutical industry in drug development. A part of his research was working with placebos alongside the drugs being tested. He was so intrigued by the extraordinary results of the placebos—sometimes better than the drugs—that he left the industry to write and speak about the power of the human mind in healing.

Placebo results are an unwelcome reality in the world of pharmaceuticals because of their incredible effectiveness. The placebo is evidence that the body heals itself with the power of belief. The |Spontaneous Remission Project[1] statistics from the Institute of Noetic Sciences is filled with cases, from MDs, of people with "fatal" illnesses who have fully recovered.

When we commit to this type of self-healing we are rewiring the brain to believe in wholeness and the regeneration of the body. We see ourselves as already healed. We focus on the intelligence within and give it a rehabilitation plan. When we do so, we are causing the body to fire off a host of healing chemicals and training the mind and body to shift into homeostasis, which is exactly what it was created to be in. Bringing the brain and the heart into coherence brings the body into coherence.

If you are interested in learning how to do this, I recommend Dr. Dispenza's books *You Are the Placebo* and *Breaking the Habit of Being Yourself.* Downloadable MP3 guided meditations and MP4 classes are available on his website. If you are able, get yourself to a workshop to properly understand the powerful potential of this work.

Through guided meditations, Dr. Joe brings us into the sweet spot of being no one, in no place, transcending time and stepping into consciousness where all things are possible. We leave the place of matter and the old stories of our mind and move into a space where we can let go and access divine wisdom. We get beyond our identity as a cancer patient and rise above our emotionally chaotic states. It takes commitment—of that there is no doubt—but it is a priceless investment of time.

Afterward, we observe our thoughts and emotions so that we do no slip into obsessing about our disease or allow despair to overtake us. We let go of analysis or predicting outcomes. Not always easy to do, but we curtail talking about the condition and dis-identify with it. We do things outside of habit and think new thoughts. We move forward and live as though our prayers have been answered and as though we are connected to a new future of health and happiness. The body may take a while to catch up to this new reality, but with diligence, changes will occur.

The first hurdle to overcome is a lack of belief. Without a level of belief, you will not be inspired to do the inner work. Any good doctor will admit that belief and faith are dynamic agents in a human being's healing.

The second challenge is summoning the determination and dedication

---

1   http://noetic.org/research/projects/spontaneous-remission/faqs

to sit in quietude and do the meditations. Basically, the process of change and self-healing has to become *the* most important thing in your life.

One would think that self-preservation would trump everything, but in my own life, I struggle to dedicate myself to the internal changes I wish to make through this process. While I was in treatment and recovery I devoted myself daily to visualization and meditation. Now, caught up in other pursuits and distractions, I procrastinate, so I understand resistance and the challenge of mustering self-motivation. But the techniques in Dr. Dispenza's guided meditations, along with daily positive self-talk, and a commitment to changing poor mental habits will only cause goodness in our lives. The resolve to heal has to come from a reservoir within.

We have all been conditioned to believe otherwise, but science is proving, beyond all doubt, how formidable our beliefs are in creating health or illness, happiness or chaos.

You are amazingly powerful.

Documentary of interest: What the Bleep do We Know!?
http://www.whatthebleep.com/

Dr. Joe Dispenza's Channel
https://www.youtube.com/user/drjoedispenza

Dr. David Hamilton's Channel
https://www.youtube.com/user/davidrhamiltonphd

The Rabbit Hole of Reinventing Yourself

"We can't solve problems by using the same kind of thinking we used when we created them."
—Albert Einstein

"As within, so without."
—Hermessianex

"It's not the load that breaks you down, it's the way you carry it."
—Lou Holtz

"Your only limitation is the one you set up in your own mind."
—Napoleon Hill

"As he thinks, so he is; as he continues to think, so he remains."
—James Allen

So what in the hell does that really mean? Delving into the new (and very exciting) world of neuroplasticity, I think I may finally—after much seeking—understand the science of how the brain works and how we can truly reinvent our personalities and our day-to-day lives.

Trying to figure out why my life is somewhat like *Groundhog Day* (the movie) has been the blight of my existence for far too long. How can someone be reasonably intelligent, creative, have business acumen, and do oodles of things to reach a dream, and still wake up each day to a lot of reoccurring experiences with only some different players? Not only has it been a mystery to me, but to friends, family, coaches, and teachers who have watched me.

I am thrilled when I see odd sparks, new little bits of magic or manna here and there, like dialing a radio and finding a favorite song on a station, but then I hit the mountains (a challenge), lose the frequency, and static returns.

First I read *The Brain that Changes Itself*. Then *How God Changes your*

Brain. I recently began immersing—and I mean submerging and steeping myself—in the work of Dr. Joe Dispenza. Finding myself in a dark night of the soul, I got to the fall-on-your-knees moment of feeling the time had come to flush or swim (to use the Fish Called Wanda analogy). I asked (okay … pleaded) for an answer, for the missing piece of this bizarre life puzzle. And I got it.

Dispenza, the popular fellow from *What the Bleep Do We Know!?* and *What the Bleep!?: Down the Rabbit Hole*, takes the quantum model, and in layman's terms, explains how we can rewire our brains to create a "redesigned" personality and subsequent new reality. It brings the law of attraction to a whole new level and answers a good part of the reason why the "law" works for some, but not others.

To take Einstein's quote above a little further, we cannot bring bold dreams to fruition, no matter how many things we do, how many affirmations we say, or how hard we try, if we are doing it with the same stale mindset in the world of matter.

Dispenza's theory is that we live in either a state of survival or a state of creation. In a state of survival, we live in reaction to our environment, which means we are at the mercy of the outer world. If shit happens, we react with a surge of emotions that batters our system. We anticipate new experiences—with jobs, lovers, friendships, family—based on what has happened in the past. When we step back as an observer of ourselves and fast from our usual emotional reactions, we have an opportunity to create anew.

Active creation comes in first realizing that a) we *do* have the power to create a much more vibrant life, b) we need to discipline ourselves to do the work involved, and c) we must nurture the fortitude to continue in faith and have the patience to await results.

If you don't believe we have that kind of power over our minds and emotions, watch the true story of *A Beautiful Mind*.

The work involved? In a simplistic nutshell:

- Spending some time before we get out of bed to set intentions for our day and to ask for help and for evidence (signs that tell us we are consciously affecting our outcomes through our intentions).

- Meditating and visualizing, or as Dispenza calls it, rehearsing a new life, daily and repetitively so that we can walk into the new without resistance from our minds or from that little devil within that says, *that'll never happen—it never has before, so give it up, dude!*

- Observing what we react to and how our body feels (when adrenaline and corrosive chemicals surge—what Eckhart Tolle calls the 'pain body') as well as catching ourselves when falling back into the painful, albeit comfortable ruts that physiologically and tangibly resides in our brains.

- Constructing new roadways by trusting and by developing new responses and exciting visions for our lives.

In this process, we are pruning away the old mind, releasing the old self, and cultivating a new personality and a fresh reality. Just as an unused path in a forest is difficult to access, so too are the trails of negativity when left ignored. The brain is a large part of the science of reinvention, but the big, indomitable heart is not left out of the equation.

As we release primitive, lower frequency emotions and are no longer enslaved by them, we liberate the energy of our divinity. When we meditate and enter our internal landscape, the heart speaks. We stop analyzing, judging, and predicting. We move from a narcissistic state to a more selfless perspective.

The grand message in all of this is that *if* your emotions and thoughts are careening down a slippery slope, detour them now. Before something brings you to your knees.

A few years back, when I was in a stressful job, I distinctly recall thinking that my recurring thoughts and bad feelings were not good for my health. I innately knew that I was harming my body, yet I could not stop myself from being sucked into the whirling dervish within.

I am not much of a bible quoter, but my favorite promise is, "I will restore to you the years the locusts have eaten." (Joel 2:25) In Catholicism I was taught to take the bible literally, which I never bought. I believe the messages are threaded with a much deeper, figurative wisdom. I now realize what the locusts actually are: fear, disappointment, doubt, anger, guilt, regret, despair, judgment, self-criticism, etc.

And I also realize that we ourselves, in co-creation with the greater mind, can restore the years that have been wasted in a state of mere survival and have left us with ill effects and residue. Our withered "crops" can be revived and miracles can abound from places we had not imagined when we tap into a new way of thinking and a solid source of power.

Is it easy?

Not.

At.

All.

I have just begun emotional rehab and I liken my addiction to emotional states and survival mode to getting off crack. One needs to be ever vigilant. Cutting through old patterns and identifying preconceived outcomes I have developed based on the past is hard work. You must "lose your mind" to develop a new one. It is time-consuming and exhausting. And, being human, I can find all kinds of diversions to keep me from sitting in contemplation. Yet when I do, cool things happen.

Is it worth it? Well, I can ask, is it loving and kind to torment yourself with nasty emotions and hanging on to past hurts? Would you rather live by rote or by creation?

The big thinkers—Martin Luther King, Mother Theresa, Nelson Mandela, Ghandi—these groundbreakers stepped away from the known and accepted norms to embrace what they believed they could change in the world in spite of all evidence to the contrary.

I guess the question is, are you worth it?

The Rabbit Hole of Reinventing Yourself
http://wp.me/p2ACw4-dH
lifebyheart.wandasthilaire.com

44

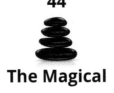

The Magical

"The world is full of magical things patiently waiting for our senses to grow sharper."
—William Butler Yeats

In Pam Grout's books E^2 (*E-Squared*) and E^3 (*E-Cubed*), she outlines simple experiments for proving that we create our reality and that we have access to the field all day, every day. She reminds us to ask: for gifts, for manna, for magic, for miracles. We can invite assistance.

If you are prone to avoiding the use of the word 'magic' and it has connotations of the occult to you, suspend your opinion. As poet Yeats said, the world is full of magical things. Serendipity, synchronicity, and coincidences transform the mundane into the magical. The wonders of nature gift us with a sparkle of enchantment.

Lorna Byrn says, in *Angels in my Hair*, that we all come with a guardian angel for life and that we can ask for help and intervention from this angel at any time. I frequently ask and invite guides and angels to assist me.

While writing this book, I sent off two separate birthday cards to my twin niece and nephew for their 16th birthday. Reviewing my day in bed before slumber, I patted myself on the back for getting them out on time. And then it dawned on me—I had put them in the post box with no postage. I asked the angels to deliver the cards in spite of the absence of stamps, a massive request if you know the Canadian Postal system. Three days later, my brother confirmed they arrived! Both envelopes went through, minus postage. I prefer to think they did so on the wings of an angel.

When was the last time you played with the divine? Whether your belief systems are based on God, Jesus, the Universe, the Force, the Quantum Matrix, the Field of Potentiality, your Higher Self, or angels and guides, *now* is the time for prayer or conversation with him, her, it, or them.

I have been speaking with the divine for most of my life and Pam's books reminded me of the fun of a playful daily practice. It is always a thrill when things come, both big and small, after I ask.

The other day I bought a bone for a client's dog and thought, *I should pop into the Goodwill next door to see if they have the book I want.* The store has a tiny reading section and the book I wanted was available in hardcover format only, so chances were slim. It was also a new, popular release about the creative process called *Big Magic* by Elizabeth Gilbert.

I danced to Michael Jackson playing in the background as I browsed. There, standing alone between two rows of books, was *Big Magic*. I let out a yelp—a pristine $30 hardcover book for $3.

This has to be angels at work. This is crazy. What are the chances? I thought.

I walked around the corner and a peculiar fellow walked towards me in a florescent orange workman's vest and matching socks.

"Hey … Hi!" he said.

"Hello!" I answered.

"This copy of *White Christmas* is rare you know," he held up a video. "It's the one where the guy tries to kill himself, but the angels come and help him. There are angels you know. They *are* real."

"Ya, I know it." I said.

He leaned in, looked me directly in the eyes with deep intensity and said, "You gotta face your fears. If you don't, they'll just chase you."

I had just been through a series of confrontations that had forced me to deal with a range of old fears. I don't know about you, but I thought that was a cool moment of big magic.

You, too, can ask for support. Request an infusion of courage, strength, and health. Ask your guardian angel to quell your fears and calm you.

Play with divinity. You are not just a weak human flailing through life alone. You are a part of a divine matrix; one that is infinite and unlimited, and you have access to all kinds of amazing magical happenstances, if only you'll just ask.

Life by Heart
Practical Everyday Magic
11/19/2013

"There are only two ways to live your life. One is as though nothing is a miracle. The other is as though everything is a miracle."
—Albert Einstein

One morning while getting ready for the day, I pondered the concept of bending reality and of adding a little more practical magic to my life. A moment later, my neighbor knocked on the door to ask if he could use my garage and said that he would bring by $150 later. In a writer's life, that's a bit of manna from heaven.

When I was a child, I believed fervently in magic. I was captivated by the idea of creating things from some secret power within. I was 11 when we moved from Saskatoon to the big city of Edmonton, and I befriended a quiet girl whose elderly parents seemed rather stodgy and their lives were as sensible and boring as one could imagine. She too was taken with the idea of magic and we toyed with the notion that we could become sorceresses (much to my sister's amusement and ridicule). It was all fun and games until we freaked ourselves out by casting a "spell" on the nincompoop who taught our Language Arts class and he came in the next day with a broken ankle.

My life has been an odd blend of crisis and magic. In spite of the many challenges I have faced, I believe myself to have good luck and the ability to create happy surprises. I have had friends ask me, "how *do* you do it?" at the times that I have manifested incredible deals, new cars, vacations, and money out of the blue when my circumstances appear quite the contrary. They do not believe me when I say it's pure magic and miracles.

I once worked for a wicked, despotic corporation. Although it was a Canadian company, my regional sales managers were always based in the USA. When my fourth manager in under two years was to come visit me, I wished and visualized him to be delayed someplace. I was tired of breaking in new managers who would inevitably leave in short order. He was waylaid and never made it to Calgary. When the fifth one was scheduled to meet me, I did the same and willed it *hard*. It was right down to the wire—Monday morning, two hours before he was to arrive at the airport—when I received a message that he had already quit! I left the job before I had to endure the next manager, but I felt like I had somehow generated a little bit of magic.

One of the hardest things for a human being to do is hold a vision of something better when shite is all that is in front of us. When we are swirling in the cesspool, we do not have the power to create from that foul space. But when we can crawl out of it and hang on to a bigger, better picture, we are able to access that sweet spot of manifestation.

The next hardest thing is remembering and disciplining ourselves to actually *do* the work, diligently. We can be somewhat lazy, especially about doing something on speculation.

We are taught that matter is solid and time unalterable. But we are now learning, as humans did when they found out that the Earth was, in fact, not flat, that the Newtonian physics we were indoctrinated with is not exactly accurate. It is the stuff we learned in our science classes and that our parents and grandparents taught us. Under those laws, life has been—for eons—very rigid, linear, and logical.

The "real" world drags us down into the illusion that we are powerless to affect and bend our reality. People will pee on your parade when you begin to think bigger than your life. I have had many a scoffing laugh at my ideas.

Looking back, the '80s and early '90s was an exceptionally carefree era. Imagine that on a flight back from Italy, I sat in the cockpit with two handsome Italian pilots drinking Campari and soda. In less than 20 years, the world has become a place where you can kiss that kind of frivolous freedom behind. But can we still inject our lives with a daily dose of magic and live in a space of more charm?

I have contemplated the idea of everyday magic a lot since a visit with my dad in Edmonton a few weeks ago. He religiously listens to a nightly radio program that delves into all types of things, but has a focus on the negative aspects of what is going on in the world, such as the scary Orwellian tactics that we do not even realize we're immersed in and the things that "they" are doing to us behind the scenes.

Even if we think we can filter and remain impervious when we watch or listen to a barrage of bad news and negativity, I don't believe we can.

What we think about, watch a lot of, or focus on has a direct effect on our reality.

So, I thought, what if I could convince my dad to do an experiment with me? What if he (and I) were to fast from this type of information and instead make a concerted effort to focus, as best as possible, on the magic, serendipity, and synchronicity in the world?

How?

Firstly, by noticing and appreciating the small miracles and gifts. They are in front of us every single day.

Secondly, by adding a dose of wonder. What would you like to experience in your life that seems a bit improbable?

I wonder ... if this job could become a dream job?
I wonder ... how could I get in better shape and enjoy it?
I wonder ... can I get to Spain this summer?
I wonder ... how my husband and I can spice up our love life?
I wonder ... how could I revitalize myself and feel awesome?

Obsess about the most wonderful thing that could happen to you. Next, just allow. Open your figurative arms to permit something fun and unexpected and a little mystical to enter. Invite magic.

Lastly, you have heard it a hundred times. Practice gratitude daily. I have been playing with the technique this extraordinary little girl uses and it's hilariously fun! *Jessica's "Daily Affirmation"*[1]

I do not say this from a Pollyanna point of view. I have had life knock me on my ass more times than I care to remember, so I know planet Earth can be a harsh place, especially in this epoch. I say this because I have learned that life is fleeting.

Whether you believe only in logic or have an inkling that there is the possibility of magic and miracles in this dimension, would you rather hunker down into a life of quiet desperation and pragmatism, or would you prefer to spend the rest of your days, weeks, months, or years with a dusting of enchantment?

When the going gets dull, the dull need a spritzing of practical magic. Life is either a bitch and then you die, or it is an opportunity to Merlin-ize. And the fun part is, we get to choose!

---

1   https://youtu.be/qR3rK0kZFkg

Practical Everyday Magic
http://wp.me/p2ACw4-j1
lifebyheart.wandasthilaire.com

45

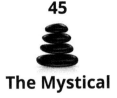

The Mystical

"Sacred signs always come when your soul calls out in pain or joy."
—Lawren Leo

I often find bizarre or precious little things on my path. And a friend asked me why I always find these treasures. It told her it is because I ask. Frequently.

One day after I told someone about my guardian angel, a few moments later I found a small metal pendant with an angel etched on it. It was on the ground in a parking lot right next to a dime. I could have used a lot more than ten cents right then, but I was elated. I turned the angel medallion over and read the inscription under the dim glow of a streetlight: *"Always with you."* It gave me goose bumps. I chose to give the discovery meaning.

It is comforting to watch for signs that lead us along our life's path. Sometimes they come in a form of an immaculate white feather or an unusual animal sighting. It may be a song or a slip of paper you find on the ground with a message. It could be something a friend mentions or a sentence from an interview you hear on the radio. Signs can be like breadcrumbs to follow and can come from anywhere. Watch and listen for them. Don't overanalyze them; simply acknowledge them when they arrive.

The divine has a sense of humor, so expect anything. Last week as I went out for a walk I asked for something in the shape of a heart to let me know if there was potential with a new love connection. I laughed aloud when I found a child's hair band with a small sparkly blue heart imprinted with the image of Olaf from *Frozen*. Olaf is innocent and outgoing and is a snowman that loves all things summer—like me. The theme song, *Let it Go*, came to mind when I found it. A few days later the love interest proved to be fickle and flakey—let it go!

It may feel silly at first, but be open to signs. We are usually too lost in the noise of our practical lives to, firstly, see them and, secondly, find meaning in them. Step past practicality and into playfulness and innocence. Dance with the divine and ask for signs along your cancer passage.

Subtle Signs and Sweet Serendipity
10/2/2014

"Life is not merely a series of meaningless accidents or coincidences, uh uh, but rather, it's a tapestry of events that culminate in an exquisite, sublime plan."
—From the movie *Serendipity*

Whether an atheist, spiritualist, Christian, Jew, Buddhist, or otherwise, people like receiving signs. Should I take the job offer? Is this the man for me? Is a trip to Greece the right thing to do now? When something jumps out at us as an obvious sign of which direction to take, or shouts at us, *"Yes! Do it!"* we feel an affirmative declaration on our decisions.

Since the dawn of intellect, humans have followed totemism and looked for signs and symbolism in religion, mythology, paganism, Native American culture, and most ancient civilizations have documented them, such as Egyptian and Mayan. Many believe that the Universe or God/gods speaks to us through signs and omens. Our personalities may want the tangible and logical, but our souls feed off of unexpected mysteries. Serendipity is defined as a fortunate happenstance or pleasant surprise that could be orchestrated by a greater mind.

The incredible success of the simple little book, *The Alchemist*, by Paulo Coelho tells me that I am not the only one who lives by signs. Celebrities from all walks have touted the value of this parable-style story in their lives. The protagonist is an Andalucian shepherd named Santiago who travels in search of treasure. The theme of the book is finding one's destiny through signs and serendipity. Weaved throughout the tale is the message, "when you want something, all the Universe conspires in helping you achieve it."

The book has sold over *65 million* copies and has been translated into more than 67 languages making Coelho the most translated living author. In May 2014 it was in its 303rd consecutive week on The New York Times Best Seller list. I'd have to say the Universe conspired in a significant way with Mr. Coelho.

When serendipity happens and you are in the right place at the right time, it feels magical. It could be a connection for the perfect job, an incredible event you stumble upon, the finding of a new best friend, or meeting the person you'll one day marry. It feels so good because you didn't have to work hard for it, it just appeared.

Of synchronicity (sister of serendipity), Deepak Chopra says, *"My own life has been touched often by synchronicity, so much so that now I get on an airplane expecting the passenger in the next seat to be surprisingly important to me, either just the voice I need to hear to solve a problem or a missing link in a transaction that needs to come together."*

I recently sent a YouTube link to my manager with a song I love by a talented, soulful singer. I thought she'd like his music. As she read my email, that same song played on the radio and was dedicated to a young mother whose husband had just left her. She called it a 'Godcidence.'

In 1990 when I was in the hospital awaiting the results of my pathology report to find out if the (breast) cancer was localized or had spread to the lymph nodes, three friends came to see me. The visit was especially emotional because the next morning was verdict day. My friend's mother had died not long before of breast cancer. Lynne gifted me a consoling little book that evening called, *If You're Afraid of the Dark, Remember the Night Rainbow.*

When the girls left, I began to cry and walked down the hall to my lonely hospital bed. An ethereal iridescent light streamed into the stark room, the type of light that occurs only occasionally and just before the dusk settles into darkness. I went to the window. There in the sky was a full, sublime night rainbow. My heart leapt and I felt that I had been sent a good omen from Lynne's mum, telling me that all would be well. The next morning the tests came back clear. I still have that book and whenever I see a night rainbow, my heart swells and I am soothed.

Have you ever asked for a sign and got one that was undeniable? We can choose to see symbolism and meaning in the seemingly random things that cross our paths or we can bypass and ignore them. In native culture there is an entire "medicine" which explains the meaning of each animal that crosses our lives. I frequently ask for signs through nature.

When I was buying my last car, the process was nerve-wracking. I was no longer working in my higher paying career and I was anxious about the approval process. Although I loved the car I'd had at the time, it was in need of a new transmission and brakes and I couldn't fix it.

Distracted with worry while awaiting word as I drove through the countryside, I said aloud, *"Okay. This is making me nuts. I just need to know if the new car is mine. Please bring me a sign through animals. Not a crow or anything common. I need an unusual sighting so I know for sure it's all going to be okay. Thank you."*

Less than five minutes later in the field to the right was a majestic moose surrounding by twelve deer! I had to turn the car around just to be sure I was seeing clearly. I stopped on the side of the road and a few of the creatures looked up at me. All of them kept grazing. I observed in awe and drove off with a Zen calmness. Three days later, that sweet new car was mine. I named her Angel Baby.

This summer I began a conversation with that most revered of masters, Jesus. I was raised Catholic, but do not follow any dogma. Two women in my life were gently pushing and I've been having a difficult time, so I decided to have a discussion with 'The Man.' I believe he existed, I believe he was who they claim he was, but I still don't grasp the insistent "you *must* accept Christ into your life" thing. And I certainly don't want to do it via a bunch of rules and pomposity.

We had a number of one-sided chats and since I didn't hear back, I asked for signs that he was listening to me. The first thing that happened was that a tattooed, pierced, hipster chick at a ticket stand for *Cavalia* softly said to me on my way out the door, "Remember, Jesus loves you."

"*What?*" I said.

"He does. Jesus loves you," she said as she smiled.

The old man standing behind me nearly fell over. She was the last person we'd have expected to hear such a comment from, especially so out of context.

The second sign was in a bar (I love the oxymoronic). My dad and I were having lunch and our pretty, belly-baring waitress had a script tattoo on her forearm in a foreign language. I asked what it said. It was in Polish and was something her grandmother had taught her. It was Revelation 21:4 and translated it read:

"God shall wipe away all tears from their eyes; and there shall be no more death, neither sorrow, nor crying, neither shall there be any more pain: for the former things are passed away."

The next thing that occurred was that one passage appeared in my life *three* times over a short period. The first appearance was a quotation at the very end of a book I was reading. The second was, once again, a tattoo. It was on the arm of a new barista at my coffee shop. The tattoo was massive, covering the distance of his whole forearm, and just read: Jeremiah 29:11. I asked him to recite it to me and realized it was the same psalm I'd seen only days before. Even though I frequent this café, I have never seen him again. Two weeks later, I received an email and in it the same psalm closed a personal message to me.

Jeremiah 29:11 reads:

"For I know the plans I have for you," declares the Lord, "plans to prosper you and not to harm you, plans to give you hope and a future."

I also found the extended New International Version 29:11-13:

"For I know the plans I have for you," declares the Lord, "plans to prosper you and not to harm you, plans to give you hope and a future. [12] Then you will call on me and come and pray to me, and I will listen to you. [13] You will seek me and find me when you seek me with all your heart."

Ironically, just after I wrote the above story I saw someone retweeted me on Twitter. His profile included—you got it—*Jeremiah 29:11.*

Coincidence? Maybe. But I don't think so.

I believe there is infinitely more to life than what we know with our five senses. Personally, I find it comforting to think someone or something is looking out for me and listening. When life is moving at warp speed or when it's all in a tidy flow, we are less likely to watch for signs.

Maybe I (and others like me) am making a mountain out of a molehill. But conversing with the unseen and asking for signs and serendipity can bring another facet to life. With the world seemingly off its rocker, we sorely need a little mysterious goodness. We need hope that there's something more. With a daily cascade of idiotic news—things like Big Pharma patenting human genes[1]—we all could use a lot more awe.

Is the Universe speaking to you through signs? Are you open to

---

1 http://www.theguardian.com/world/2014/sep/05/
court-rules-breast-cancer-gene-brca1-patented-australia

looking or listening for them? If you poopoo a series of "coincidences," are you dismissing the wondrous?

I challenge you to suspend disbelief for the next week and ask for/look for signs. Watch for unusual things in nature. Pay attention to interesting happenstances. Expect the unexpected.

As poet David Whyte says, "Your great mistake is to act the drama as if you were alone."

Subtle Signs and Sweet Serendipity
http://wp.me/p2ACw4-rQ
lifebyheart.wandasthilaire.com

46

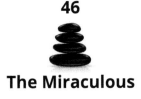

The Miraculous

"Be realistic: Plan for a miracle."
—Osho Rajneesh

I heard Anita Moorjani speak on Dr. Oz about how she has been accused of giving cancer patients "false hope." I loved her response.

She said, "What's worse? Giving people hope for surviving cancer or a doctor using his human capacity to predict someone's life span and planting the seed of imminent death?"

One thing that endlessly surprises me is when people would rather choose not to believe in miracles and magic than to opt in. The world is brimming with stories of Eleventh Hour miracles of every conceivable form.

I came into life believing. I have been forever fascinated by the manifestation of miracles. Society does everything it can to hammer that notion out of us. We have all been advised, through our culture, our families, our friends, our teachers, and our religions, how we must face the reality of "what is" and live in rationality.

The cool thing? "What is" can change instantaneously.

Right now, as you traverse the rocky landscape of Cancerland, tales of incredible miracles may sound pretty pie-in-the-sky. But do you remember times when you met the right person at the perfect time? Or an unexpected gift came to you out of nowhere? Or money came in at the final hour to save the day? We can ask for miracles.

There was the day I sat at a red light in the midst of my second cancer journey awaiting surgery. Having lost my job, therefore having no benefits, I was obsessing over my bills. As I fretted, a question popped in my mind: *can you trust that it will work out?* I relaxed and acquiesced. *I will trust,* I told myself and stopped the stinking thinking.

Ten minutes later, my friend Shari called to ask me if I was feeling lucky.

"Not particularly," I said.

"Well you should be because you just won the 50/50 for the studio fundraiser!"

"Seriously? No way!"

"Way! $4400! Cash."

That money miracle covered my bills for the next couple of months.

Many years earlier I had a markedly poignant moment in Mexico on the beach that I shall never, ever forget. My husband and I were newly separated after a painful, but necessary, ultimatum. Following this I had booked the trip with two close friends to help ease my agonizing heartbreak. Just prior to the flight to Mexico, my back went into spasm so badly I couldn't get out of bed or walk without assistance. The pain was excruciating.

My chiropractor made a house call and gently informed me I was having hysterical paralysis caused by the shock of the break-up. He said it was genuine physical paralysis which was like a vise grip on my spinal cord and that I should try my best to relax.

We kept our plans to go, but I was not an easy travel mate. The girls had to carry me everywhere and I whimpered in my sleep all night long from the pain. One morning the two wanted to go for a long walk along the beach. They dragged me down to the ocean and set me under an umbrella at a beachfront café. After they left, tears streamed down my face. I was in inconceivable physical pain, but to make matters worse, I was emotionally devastated. The waiter didn't know what to think and asked if there was anything at all that he could do for me.

Left alone staring out at the ocean I made a simple, gut-wrenching statement aloud:

God must not live in Mexico. I could not possibly be in this much pain if he did.

The next moment, everything went still. The birds that had been squawking were mute and the waves stopped. I heard no people—only silence. Then I heard one short sentence:

Yes, he does.

The sounds of life returned and the waves lapped the shore. I sat dumbfounded.

Did I really hear that? Am I going crazy from the grief and back pain?

The next morning, I awoke completely pain free. I stood up and walked as though nothing was ever wrong. I could not believe it. The girls were stunned. Guests at the pool who had seen me in a back brace being carried about appeared mystified as I strolled by. I knew I had experienced a miracle.

There is no such thing as false hope. Hope is hope. My underlying mission with this book is to incite a sense of miracles and the impossible becoming possible. Wet blanket people are a dime a dozen. Veer away from them and place your precious self into a cocoon of the miraculous.

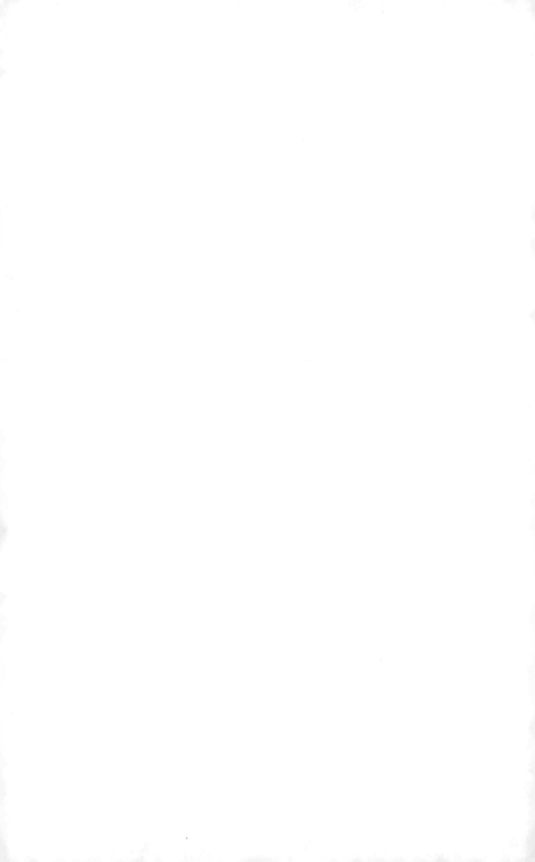

47

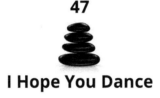

I Hope You Dance

"People will do anything, no matter how absurd, to avoid facing their own souls."
—Carl Jung

It might seem that the easiest thing to do in life is go through it in a state of unconsciousness. As Dr. Bruce Lipton often says, the movie *The Matrix* is actually a documentary; we live in an illusory world and can take the red pill or the blue. You choose.

Oftentimes we feel like the victim of some bizarre scheme, as though we are randomly handed mayhem and chaos and that we must plod from one challenge to the next. We cannot control the storms that hit our lives, but we can control our thoughts and actions.

Our feelings are frequently derived from judgment calls about our circumstances—happy or sad—rather than from a steady inner strength that is not swayed by events. I am still a fledgling; although I understand this at an intellectual level, persuasive emotions and the roadmaps of the past still hijack me. Old tapes fight to win and often do. And it takes vigilance to create my life rather than react to it.

What I have come to learn through copious challenges, obstacles, and roadblocks is that life responds to us. We are connected to a field that is malleable and eavesdrops on what we think, speak, and feel. Instead of taking it personally, we can consider the idea that our life is an expression of the "frequency" we are resonating at and that at any moment we have the power to change it to a new upper octave.

Is it easy?

No. None of the changes I have outlined are—because of the way we have been conditioned. But in a Kaizen, bit-by-bit approach, they are achievable with the ultimate goal of health and happiness.

I hope you have given great contemplation to your inner world. If you are being harsh with yourself, if you have an internal slave driver with a metaphorical whip pushing you to be better and do more, my wish is that you have given it a pink slip from your life.

We have been on quite a sojourn together, you and I. As aforementioned, this work was assigned to me, not by a publisher or editor, but by Spirit. On a cold November morning I was given orders; I did not chase this mission, it chased me.

Once I wrote the first outline of the book, I worked for 18 months, everyday, sometimes into the wee hours—not at the directive of anyone, but of my own volition. I dug deeply into the well of my experiences, many very painful, and sifted through all that I have learned from an array of brilliant leaders, scientists, and masters.

I have endeavored to bring you valid and pertinent information to help you make the best decisions. As much as I value truth and abhor injustice, I have spent my life veering away from controversy and avoiding confrontation, so this has been a wild, scary leap into the abyss.

As I go further and further down the rabbit hole with this undertaking, my heart keeps expanding for you, and for humanity at large. I have never been a mother—nor had the instinct—but through this work, I feel a deep calling to bring comfort and to be a messenger for a world so very tired.

I want you to heal. I want you to thrive. And I want you to give yourself permission to be as real and as authentically *you* as you have ever been; to laugh when you want to; to cry when you need to; to be angry at God if you are; to forgive yourself—and everyone—fully; to feel free to make mistakes; to tell your truth; to see your incredible beauty; to seek your own unique brand of joy; to be vulnerable; to take a stand; to rest; to dream; to own your purpose; to live in magic and allow miracles; to let go; to start anew. I hope that this work lifts your spirits and supports you to love and believe in yourself. I want you to know in the core of your being that you are loved.

As you make this passage and move onward, instead of diving headfirst into endless goals and burdensome tasks, ponder the idea of imposing a new, improved signature on the canvas of your life. Ignore what others are doing. Fall in love with life and yourself and be your own hero in your cancer journey, no matter the outcome.

Life is crazy and keeps getting crazier. The world we knew no longer exists and a new way of healing is rapidly emerging. We can live in fear and contract into confusion and complaint, or we can look at the new discoveries and doctrinal shifts with excitement and anticipation.

Because of my unceasing fascination for the human potential, I study this daily. People shatter paradigms every day. "Inexplicable" healings and spontaneous remissions occur the world over. Impossible records are broken. Humans overcome the unimaginable. And the wonderful part is that once someone breaks an old, worn out belief about what we are capable of, it gives us all permission to follow suit—the 100th monkey, so to speak.

At the 2016 Tony Awards, winner Frank Langella said: *"When something bad happens, we have three choices. We can let it define us, we can let it destroy us, or we can let it strengthen us."* Cancer can define us if we let it, it can destroy us, but it can also strengthen us in ways we would never have imagined when we first were handed the diagnosis.

I wholly acknowledge that we cannot bend everything to our will. We are humans and humans break. Unfortunately pain is a part of life and it is not always easy. There is still great mystery in the way life unfolds and the plan may be preset; we cannot know. But we can keep aspiring to understand ourselves and to live fully until we leave.

I believe love is the unifying field that connects the Universe based on my own personal experiments, experiences, and subsequent evidence. Keep your heart open wide—love can move mountains. Let go, breathe, and enjoy this gorgeous planet to the full, in spite of this unexpected detour.

Laugh more, work less.
Play.
Let nature be your sanctuary.
Love deeply.
Live in awe.

And I hope you dance.

My Gratitude

A million thank yous to my soul sister editor Marie Beswick-Arthur and to Ryan Fitzgerald for your good work helping me to birth this book into reality. Thank you Dianne Quinton, for pushing me forward on this project with cheerleader-style encouragement and a firm hand.

I wish to acknowledge the doctors who, at one time or another, have been in service to me through my journey and have shown me incredible care, kindness, and patience. I tip my hat in gratitude to Dr. Lindskoog, Dr. Starreveld, Dr. Cumming, Dr. Trotter, Dr. Romo, Dr. Kish, Dr. Lobay, and the amazing women who work at and manage the Breast Cancer Supportive Care Foundation in Calgary.

With all of my heart, I thank the wise women healers who have guided me, taught me, and healed me with exemplary compassion and astounding generosity: Erin Taylor, Christine Brennan, Bert Enns, Mari Torres, Maraya Edwards, Terry Kohl, Selena Murillo, Danielle Belanger, and again, Dianne Quinton—all beautiful souls.

I don't know if I can ever repay my family and friends for your fierce and all- encompassing support and TLC, but I hope so. I love you all to the moon and back.

I thank you, my reader, for trusting me with your cancer journey.

Thank you to the Kelly Shires Breast Cancer Foundation[1] and the Wings of Hope Breast Cancer Foundation[2], two organizations run by dedicated volunteers who work hard to truly make a difference.

This is a guidebook to navigate prevention, as much as it is for those diagnosed with disease. It is for the young and the old alike. It is designed to help people make dearly needed detours to a long, happy life. My wish is that this book finds its way into the hands of the healthy too, so that they stay well and flourish. Please share it with your loved ones.

I would be honored and most appreciative to you for a brief review on Amazon.

♥

---

1   http://www.kellyshiresfoundation.org/
2   https://www.wings-of-hope.com/

The Reinvent Cancer Project

I'm on a mission. In conjunction with my book, *What To Do After "I'm sorry, it's cancer."* I want to give people permission to navigate cancer intuitively. My objective is to reduce stress and suffering in the world. I want people to survive cancer and discover a new and improved life post-disease—to come home to their authentic self.

Phase I
Educate & Empower

Raise consciousness and awareness

- Educate and empower by getting the book into the hands of those newly diagnosed.
- Coordinate availability of the book to health and wellness professionals, and placement into libraries.
- Promote healing with the help of holistic integrative therapies.
- Incite shifts in emotional habits and patterns that will diminish stress and disease.
- Inspire people to make lifestyle changes and look at cancer in a new way.

Phase II
Embody

Mindful application of the knowledge

- Inform and educate through social media and by speaking and spreading the word.
- Form partnerships with individuals and groups whose aim is to reinvent the cancer journey.
- Continued study, research, and interviews to share.

- Develop workshops and online courses with creative solutions for wellness and happiness.
- Teach prevention through stress reduction and natural, life-affirming concepts.
- Show people how to liberate themselves to lighten up, live bigger, and love deeper.

Phase III
Endow

Philanthropic work for cancer patients in need

- Fund healing trips.
- Gift grants for holistic treatments.
- Match grants offered by other private foundations for living expenses.
- Offer scholarships for workshops.
- Cover initial cancer coaching sessions.
- Donate books.

If this book and mission resonate, please contemplate becoming a sponsor of this project. You can learn more about both at:

www.imsorryitscancer.com/reinventcancerproject

Resources

Making Lifestyle Changes that Stick

The most effective tool I have discovered concerning how to make changes in my life—small shifts that are having a big impact—is with Mel Robbin's 5 second technique. It's crazy simple, but powerful. It can help you make positive changes for your health and overall wellbeing, be it with diet, exercise, smoking, or anxiety. It's a valuable practice for all areas of life. I've had some serious procrastination issues since cancer II and I can tell you, it *works*.

I highly recommend watching Mel Robbins on her Why Motivation is Garbage[1] interview with Tom Bilyeu

Also her popular TEDxSF Talk, How to Stop Screwing Yourself Over[2].

And for a deeper understanding and scads of testimonies you can find her book, *The 5 Second Rule*, on Amazon.

Books

Spirituality and Self-Healing

- *You Can Heal Your Life*, Louise L. Hay
- *You are the Placebo: Making Your Mind Matter*, Dr. Joe Dispenza
- *Breaking the Habit of Being Yourself*, Dr. Joe Dispenza
- *The Biology of Belief*, Bruce Lipton
- *The Divine Matrix*, Gregg Braden
- *The Spontaneous Healing of Belief*, Gregg Braden
- *The HeartMath Solution*, Doc Childre and Howard Martin
- *The Brain That Changes Itself*, Norman Doidge, M.D.
- *How God Changes the Brain*, Andrew Newberg M.D.
- *Creative Visualization*, Shakti Gawain
- *How to Make the Impossible Possible*, Dr. Robert Anthony
- *A Return to Love*, Marianne Williamson

1 http://tinyurl.com/mjqpkcj
2 http://tinyurl.com/qhxtcxo

- *The Magical Path*, Marc Allen
- *Why Kindness is Good for You*, Dr. David Hamilton
- *The Seat of the Soul*, Gary Zukav
- *Power of Now*, Ekhart Tolle
- *The Tapping Solution*, Nick Ortner
- *The Magic of Thinking Big*, David Schwartz
- *The Dynamic Laws of Healing*, Katherine Ponder
- *Conversations with God*, Neale Donald Walsch
- *The Game of Life*, Florence Scovel Shinn
- *The Emotion Code*, Dr. Bradley Nelson
- *The Twelve Conditions of a Miracle*, Todd Michael
- *Power vs. Force*, Dr. David R. Hawkins
- *Tao Te Ching*, Lao Tzu
- *Who Would You Be Without Your Story?*, Byron Katie

Cancer and Wellness

- *Dying to be Me*, Anita Moorjani
- Radical Remission: Surviving Cancer Against All Odds[1], Dr. Kelly Turner
- *Anticancer: A New Way of Life*, David Servan-Shreiber
- *A Woman's Guide to Healing Breast Cancer*, Nan Lu
- *Anatomy of an Illness*, Norman Cousins
- *Quantum Healing: Exploring the Frontiers of Mind Body Medicine*, Deepak Chopra
- *N of 1, One Man's Harvard-documented remission of incurable cancer using only natural methods*, Glenn Sabin
- *Superfoods: The Food and Medicine of the Future*, David Wolfe
- *Kicking Cancer*, Rebecca Woodland (recipes and nutrition)

Inspirational

- *The Art of Doing Nothing*, Véronique Vienne
- *The Art of Growing Up: Simple Ways to Be Yourself at Last*, Véronique Vienne
- *The Alchemist*, Paulo Coelho

---

1 https://youtu.be/PX0oeUuKDjU

- *The Artist's Way* (Creativity and Journaling), Julia Cameron
- *Hidden Messages in Water*, Masaru Emoto
- *The Healing Power of Water*, Masaru Emoto
- *E² (E-Squared)* and *E³ (E-Cubed)*, Pam Grout
- *The Blue Zones*, Dan Buettner

Videos

- Cancer: The Forbidden Cures
- The Truth About Cancer (series), Ty Bollinger
- What the BLEEP Do We Know!?
- What the BLEEP!?: Down the Rabbit Hole
- I Am, Tom Shadyac
- The Shocking Truth About Your Health[1], Dr. Lissa Rankin (YouTube)
- Is There Scientific Proof You Can Heal Yourself[2], Dr. Lissa Rankin (YouTube)
- Louise Hay You Can Heal Your Life (The Movie)[3]

YouTube Channels of Interest

- FitLifeTV with Drew Canole (Health and fitness)
- Tom Bilyeu of Impact Theory (Deep personal development)
- Inspire Nation with host Michael Sandler (Personal growth, health, and motivation)
- Infinite Waters Diving Deep with Ralph Smart (Inspiration)

Life Coaching

Dianne Quinton (My amazing life coach)
dianne@theoptimalyou.com
www.theoptimalyou.com

---

1   https://youtu.be/7tu9nJmr4Xs
2   https://youtu.be/LWQfe__fNbs
3   http://www.hayhouse.com/you-can-heal-your-life-the-movie-landing

About the Author

Wanda St. Hilaire is a two-time breast cancer survivor with a predilection for research and a passion for delving into the psychology of wellness.

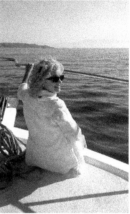

After a second diagnosis in 2010, she made lifestyle changes that contributed to her healing and supported her philosophy that our lives are meant to be lived doing what we love in places that make our hearts sing.

Through writing, St. Hilaire shares what she's learned through the high peaks of adventure and love and from the dark valleys of illness and heartbreak. Her mission is to help people overcome the self and tap into their wise inner guidance system. Her wish is to inspire others to live true to their unique and beautiful nature.

Never forget ... *impossible things happen every day.*

https://www.facebook.com/imsorryitscancer/
@spicytraveler
https://www.pinterest.com/wandasthilaire/

Other books by Wanda St. Hilaire

The Cuban Chronicles: A True Tale of Rascals, Rogues, and Romance
Of Love … Life … and Journeys
A New Life – A New Baby Boy
A New Life – A New Baby Girl
Graduate – A Little Roadmap to Your Dreams
My Love…
To You My Friend
For Your Marriage I Wish…
Newly Single Woman – A Celebration of Freedom
Newly Single Man A Celebration of Freedom
Illness – A Small Book of Comfort
The Mourning After – A Small Book of Healing

www.imsorryitscancer.com
Other books: www.writewaycafe.com
Blog: lifebyheart.wandasthilaire.com

*Your free downloadable Wellness & Self-Care Planner
is available at:*
http://imsorryitscancer.com/self-care

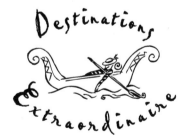

Books to incite impassioned odysses through life.

CPSIA information can be obtained
at www.ICGtesting.com
Printed in the USA
LVHW03s1711071018
592736LV00010B/690/P